£27.50

01

2

Fundamentals of Manual Therapy

Dedicated to Tsafi and the children, Mattan and Guy

Illustrations by Eyal Lederman

Eyal Lederman runs courses on manual therapy at the Centre
for Professional Development in Osteopathy and Manual
Therapy, 7 Arkansas House, New Orleans Walk, London
N19 3SZ, UK. Tel: 0171 263 8551
Fax: 0171 263 6912

For Churchill Livingstone

Editorial director: Mary Law
Project Manager: Valerie Burgess
Project development editor: Dinah Thom
Design direction: Judith Wright
Project controller: Pat Miller
Copy editor: Carrie Walker
Indexer: Tarrant Ranger Indexing Agency
Sales promotion executive: Hilary Brown

Fundamentals of Manual Therapy

Physiology, Neurology and Psychology

Eyal Lederman

Director, The Centre for Professional Development in Osteopathy and Manual Therapy, London, UK

Forewords by

Alan C. Breen DC PhD
Research Director, Anglo-European College of Chiropractic, Bournemouth, UK

Laurie S. Hartman DO MRO PhD
Associate Professor of Osteopathic Technique, British School of Osteopathy, London, UK

Dianne J. Newham MCSP PhD
Head of Physiotherapy, King's College, London, UK

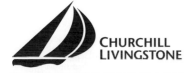

CHURCHILL
LIVINGSTONE

NEW YORK EDINBURGH LONDON MADRID MELBOURNE SAN FRANCISCO TOKYO 1997

CHURCHILL LIVINGSTONE
Medical Division of Pearson Professional Limited

Distributed in the United States of America by Churchill
Livingstone, 650 Avenue of the Americas, New York, N.Y.
10011, and by associated companies, branches and
representatives throughout the world.

First published 1997

ISBN   0 443 05275 1 8

British Library Cataloguing in Publication Data
A catalogue record for this book is available from the British
Library.

Library of Congress Cataloging in Publication Data
A catalog record for this book is available from the Library
of Congress.

Note
Medical knowledge is constantly changing. As new
information becomes available, changes in treatment,
procedures, equipment and the use of drugs become
necessary. The author and the publishers have, as far as it is
possible, taken care to ensure that the information given in
this text is accurate and up to date. However, readers are
strongly advised to confirm that the information, especially
with regard to drug usage, complies with latest legislation
and standards of practice.

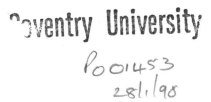

The
publisher's
policy is to use
**paper manufactured
from sustainable forests**

Printed in Great Britain by The Bath Press, Bath

Contents

Chiropractic foreword

Opening one's mind to the viewpoints of a parallel profession is always useful. For practitioners of the art of manipulation, it is nothing less than essential if patients are to benefit from the removal of tribal barriers that have stood for far too many years. This book finds a common ground to which all practitioners of manual therapy will relate, namely the body's physiological response to intervention.

Readers from a chiropractic background will find that this book has more in common with Karel Lewit's *Manipulation Therapy in Rehabilitation of the Motor System* than with A E Homewood's *Neurodynamics of the Vertebral Subluxation*, as the book takes a general view of manipulation technique and is refreshingly devoid of 'neurospeak'. The text is composed in a simple thematic way, which will have appeal to readers at all levels, including physiologists who are attempting to understand the effects of manipulation and the propositions made about them by practitioners. The visceral effects of manual therapy are put very gently and authoritatively into perspective, exposing the folly of the old vitalistic theories and replacing them with newer and richer explanations of how the many beneficial effects of manipulation *might* come about.

Readers of a more mechanistic leaning will be reminded by this text of the psychosomatic effects of manual practice, which are not to be ignored. The reader will also enjoy the reconciliation of the viewpoints of traditional rehabilitation practice with those of practice based mainly on manual skills. While the osteopathic flavour is unmistakable, Eyal Lederman's contribution to understanding is welcome and timely.

Alan C. Breen DC PhD
Research Director, Anglo-European College of
Chiropractic

Osteopathic foreword

The art and science of osteopathy is based on the ideas of one man who had a vision that has been progressively developed since the 1870's into a logical and effective system. The logic of the approach has been obvious to those working with it, and the simplicity of the system has enabled many to emulate it, with varying degrees of success. To the scientific mind, the logic may have been less than clear, and some may have considered certain aspects of the methods to be based on dogma and tradition rather than a reasoned and tried and tested thinking. Eyal Lederman has taken it upon himself to challenge many of the traditional ideas and test them against modern thinking. Where he has found them wanting, he has researched extensively and discovered several 'new truths'. This is very brave in osteopathic circles, where new ideas have often been treated with suspicion as they might be responsible for causing the system to be in some way diluted. The new wave of practitioners who have a much more scientific base to their education are probably more likely to applaud this than are some traditionalists. However, if the traditionalist is prepared carefully to digest the subject matter of this book, he or she will find that it gives many verifications for traditional methods, if not the historical thinking behind them.

There are many ways of considering the changes produced in the body by osteopathic treatment; the division of this text into local tissue response, neurological and motor system response, and psychological response allows each to be considered separately. The body is, however, always thought of as a whole, and this is clear in the body of the text.

We know that osteopathic treatment works. Maybe we will now have a different understanding of how and why it works. We may also be in a better position to adapt our methods and thinking when we are unable to adjust the approach to one that produces the required results. I am honoured and delighted to have been given the opportunity to contribute this Foreword, and hope to see further work based on this thinking to push back the frontiers of communication and thinking for the benefit of our patients.

Laurie S. Hartman DO MRO PhD
Associate Professor of Osteopathic Technique
British School of Osteopathy, UK

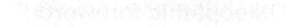

Physiotherapy foreword

Manual therapy has been practised for centuries. Over time, it has evolved to incorporate many disciplines and theories, many of which have been in conflict for at least part of their history. In recent years, there has been a growing acceptance that no single group is likely to have a monopoly on truth and that each can learn from others.

The different schools of thought have grown organically and are, for the most part, based on belief rather than knowledge. The relatively new spirit of cooperation is coupled with an acknowledgement of the need for evaluation and a move towards evidence-based practice that offers the best outcome for patients and clients. In order for this to happen, practitioners need to have a sound knowledge of a number of basic subjects, coupled with an extensive body of information in clinical and applied areas. Practitioners from all manual therapy professions are relative newcomers to research and are subject to the normal human tendency to operate within a fairly narrow band of knowledge and practice.

This book comprehensively brings together basic knowledge required by manual therapists. It also describes what is, and is not, known about the effects of manual therapy in a manner that is conducive to optimizing practice, and highlights the areas that require further basic and applied research. It is a valuable text for all those involved in any aspect of manual therapy.

Dianne J. Newham MCSP PhD
Head of Physiotherapy,
King's College, London, UK

Preface

The text and drawings of this book started out as students' notes for an undergraduate course on The Physiological Basis of Osteopathic Technique at the British School of Osteopathy. However, the search for the physiological basis of manual therapy started long before, when I was examining osteopathic harmonic techniques. I found that the physiological foundations of manual therapy were poorly understood, researched and documented. Single studies and texts gave a very patchy picture of the physiology of manual therapy. Information on why and how different techniques work and when to use them was severely lacking, a failure limited not just to my own discipline of osteopathy. In order to understand the whole phenomenon of manual therapy, I thus developed a model – the physiological model of manual therapy – which describes the physiological basis of the various manual techniques.

Understanding the physiological basis for technique is of paramount importance to the practitioner. To influence the patient's condition effectively, manual techniques must obey the physiological rules that underlie repair, healing and well-being. Understanding these rules can make manual techniques more effective and safe, as well as increase the practitioner's technique repertoire and the range of conditions that can be treated.

Manual therapy is seen as a therapeutic modality used by members of various disciplines, such as osteopaths, chiropractors, physiotherapists, etc. Manual therapists are encouraged to use all manual techniques, even those which are traditionally outside their own discipline: the most effective techniques can be used to facilitate the patient's health, regardless of the practitioner's discipline. Interdisciplinary barriers can be crossed and information shared, all with the single aim of improving the quality of treatment given to the patient.

Writing this book has dramatically changed the way in which I practise osteopathy. Some knowledge was painful to assimilate as it completely overturned many of my fundamental beliefs. However, such knowledge allowed me to expand my repertoire of techniques and treat a range of conditions that I had not previously treated. It also gave me a better sense of conviction and depth in my work. I am now more able to visualize what is happening under my hand as if I can observe the patient's interior; I can now visualize repair processes, whereas before I could only visualize structure.

The contents of this book are a great physiological puzzle. Some parts are known and some parts need to be filled in, hopefully by further research. This book by no means claims to know it all: information and knowledge is forever changing. At the beginning of my courses, I tell the students that the information is there to form a baseline from which we can communicate. I hope that this book will serve as a common baseline for the different manual disciplines, from which we can communicate with each other in a better way and find common grounds for research, all with the ultimate purpose of offering the patient better treatment.

I hope this book will convey some of the richness of manual therapy and allow the practitioner to unleash the full potency of this therapeutic modality.

London 1996   E. L.

Acknowledgements

I would like to acknowledge the following individuals who helped in the writing of this book.

Tsafi Schectman-Lederman for co-writing Section 3.

For their assessment and criticism of content: Section 1, Professor Dianne Newham, King's College, London, Dr Martin Collins, British School of Osteopathy, London; Section 2, Dr Peter Greenwood, Homerton Hospital, London, Dr John Rothwell, Queen's Hospital for Neurology, London, Professor Dianne Newham; Section 3, Tsafi Schectman-Lederman, Dr Peter Randell, Clover Southwell and Nathan Bevis.

For the photographs in Chapter 15, Anna Sherbany.

For criticism of all parts about pain mechanisms, Professor Patrick Wall, St Thomas Hospital, London.

For proofreading the text and for his kind help with all the references, Will Podmore, Librarian, British School of Osteopathy.

And to all the individuals above, and friends who helped to proofread some parts of the text.

1

Introduction

Manipulation is defined by *Dorland's Pocket Medical Dictionary* as 'skilful or dextrous treatment by the hands.' The word 'therapy' is derived from the Greek *therapeuein*, meaning 'to take care of', *'therapon'* meaning 'an attendant', a living person. 'Therapeutic' signifies the curative and healing potential of one person towards another.[1] Manual therapy is therefore the use of the hands in a curative and healing manner, and can be defined as the use of manipulation with therapeutic intent.

Manipulation is a therapeutic modality. It is not limited to the traditional users of manual therapy, such as physiotherapists, osteopaths, chiropractors and massage therapists. It includes such professionals as nurses, who use touch in nurturing premature infants or massage in supporting the terminally ill. It also includes psychotherapists, who may use touch as a therapeutic modality in encouraging client self-exploration or initiating emotional processes, and social workers or counsellors, who may use touch as support for the bereaved.

Techniques are the therapeutic tools of the manual therapist. A wealth of techniques with an understanding of their physiological basis allows for greater flexibility in treating a wide range of conditions. Understanding the mechanisms that underlie the body's physiological response to manipulation will help the practitioner to match the most suitable and effective technique to the patient's condition. This will help the patient and therapist in several ways:

- safer treatment
- more effective treatment
- reduction in the overall duration of treatment.

The purpose of this book is to discuss the possible physiological mechanisms underlying manual techniques.

The book is divided into four main sections. The first three sections are related to the three physiological organizations described above. Section 1 relates to the effect of manipulation on local tissue organization. Section 2 examines the neurophysiological aspects of manipulation, in particular the neurological organization of the motor system and neurological pain mechanisms. The autonomic nervous system is discussed in Section 3, which describes the effect of touch and manipulation on the psychological organization. Section 4 is an overview and summary of the previous three sections. Whereas in Chapters 2–4 the whole person is compartmentalized and fragmented. Section 4 aims to 'remedy' this by integrating the contents of the previous three sections and discussing their possible clinical application.

PHYSIOLOGICAL MODEL OF MANIPULATION

The aim of manual therapy is to influence the reparative and healing capacity of the individual. Change may occur at different levels in the whole person, some changes being related to local repair processes, others to improved neuromuscular function, and still others to the overall behaviour of the individual. The question arises of what makes one form of manipulation effective for reparative processes but another for neuromuscular rehabilitation. It must be assumed that different techniques will have a particular effect on certain physiological mechanisms. To illustrate these differences in response, a physiological model has been developed in which the body is arranged into three broad organizations (Fig. 1.1)[2].

- local tissue organization

- neurological organization
- psychophysiological organization.

Each level of organization will respond differently to manipulation, but only some specific forms of manipulation will affect any one of the organizations. How manipulation can be made specifically to target each organization is the basis of this book.

Local tissue organization

Basically, this level considers what happens to the tissues directly under the therapist's hands and how tissues respond to different forms of manipulation. The tissues in this organization are skin, muscles, tendons, ligaments, joint structures and different fluid systems, such as vascular, lymphatic and synovial (these will be collectively termed 'soft tissues'). The mechanical forces transmitted by the manipulation will influence the tissues in three principle ways:

1. in reparative processes following tissue damage
2. in changes in the physical and mechanical properties of tissues, for example tissue elongation/compression, elasticity, stiffness and strength
3. by local changes in tissue fluid dynamics (blood, lymph, extracellular and synovial fluids).

This section of the book examines how specific forms of manipulation can effectively influence each of these local processes. It will also examine the possible role of manipulation in affecting tissue pain processes.

Neurological organization

Although the therapist's hands are placed on distinct anatomical sites, manipulation may have more remote influences on different neurological processes. There are three areas of neurology that the manual therapist aims to influence, the most frequently considered being the motor system and pain (sensory) organization. This

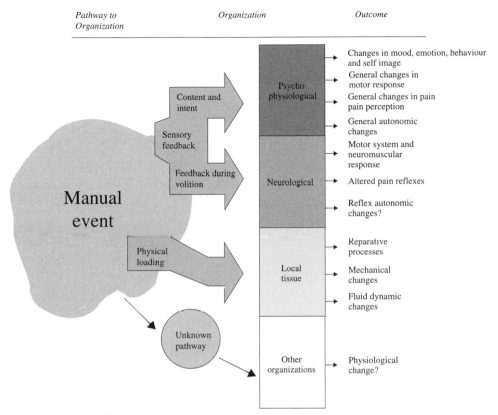

Figure 1.1   The physiological model of manipulation.

section examines how manual therapy can be used to effect neurological processes in different conditions:

- for guidance in rehabilitation of central nervous damage
- in treatment of neuromuscular deficits following musculoskeletal injury
- for postural and movement guidance
- in pain management.

There are also claims that the autonomic system may be affected by manipulation at a spinal reflex level.

Psychophysiological organization

The effects of manipulation and touch on mind and emotion play an important but often forgotten part in the overall healing process of patients. Touching the patient is seen as potent stimulus to psychological processes, but the influences of touch may not end there. Every emotion is associated with a patterned somatic response, which may manifest itself as non-specific, generalized changes in muscle tone, generalized autonomic changes and altered pain tolerance, these being only some of the whole-person responses that may be observed in the patient following manual therapy.

This division into the three organizations is somewhat artificial, as any single form of manipulation will probably affect all three organizational levels. Yet, this division is not without its purpose: it is likely that certain groups of techniques are inherently more effective than others at a particular level of organization. This inherent effectiveness has a very important clinical implication when the practitioner has to match the most effective manual technique with the patient's condition. For example, manual techniques aimed at restoring the range of movement of a joint (local tissue organization) are substantially different from those aimed at promoting general body relaxation (psycho-physiological organization). Those used for relaxation may not be effective for improving the range of movement, and vice versa. If all techniques were equally effective at all levels, it would not be necessary to have a variety of techniques: in theory, one form of manipulation would treat all conditions. Usually (but not always), most practitioners have a wide variety of techniques, and the question arises of how are these selected and matched to the patient's complaint. This book aims to clarify and offer practical models that will enhance this matching process.

Other organizational levels

There may possibly exist other organizational levels and related physiological responses, which may be affected by manipulation in a way that currently cannot be described or explained in scientific or physiological terms. For example, the concept of meridians and bioenergy forms an important part of certain manual disciplines, such as Shiatsu and Do-In. These levels of organization are outside the scope of this book but are included in this section to give a complete working model.

PATHWAYS TO THE ORGANIZATIONAL LEVELS

There are different pathways by which manipulation will 'infiltrate' the three organizational levels. At a local tissue level, the pathway is the direct mechanical loading of the tissue by manual forces. The gateway to the neurological organization is somewhat different. It is through the stimulation of proprioceptors and the use of cognition and voluntary movement. The pathway to the psychophysiological organization is also the sensory pattern evoked by the communicative or expressive content of the therapist's touch/manipulation.

REFERENCES

1. Weber R 1984 Philosophers on touch. In: Brown C C (ed.) The many faces of touch. Johnson & Johnson Baby Products Company Pediatric Round Table Series, no. 10, p 101–106

The effect of manipulation on the tissue organization

Introduction to Section 1

This Section looks at what happens to tissues that are directly under the therapist's hands, this level of work being called tissue organization. It will examine the relationship between the type of manipulation used and the eventual physiological response in the tissue. At the level of tissue organization, manipulation is seen to have several therapeutic roles (Fig. 2.1):

- To facilitate the repair processes following injury – Soft tissue injuries such as joint sprains or muscle damage are often treated by manual therapy. Normal tissue regeneration and remodelling depend on mechnical stimulation during the repair process. This mechanical environment can be provided by different forms of manipulation. This may help improve the tissue's overall mechanical and physical behaviour, such as tensile strength and flexibility.
- To affect the structure of the tissue – Soft tissue shortening can be seen in different conditions such as contractures and adhesions following tissue damage. Soft tissue shortening is often seen following central nervous system damage, e.g. stroke, or long-term adaptive postural changes. Manipulation can be used in many of these conditions to stretch and elongate the shortened tissues, improving the range of movement and reducing abnormal stresses on the body.
- To affect fluid dynamics in the tissue – The viability, health and repair of tissue are highly dependent on their vascular and lymphatic

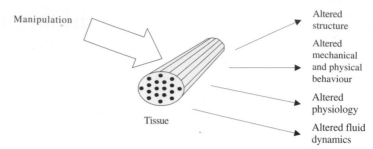

Figure 2.1 The tissue response to manipulation.

supply. This supply is important, in particular, following soft tissue damage, where there is an increased metabolic demand during repair. Manipulation may facilitate flow to and away from the tissue, improve the cellular environment and support the repair process. Its effect on fluid dynamics may also help reduce pain by encouraging the removal of inflammatory by-products and reducing tissue oedema. This role of manipulation in stimulating flow is also important in affecting synovial flow and joint repair processes. It may help reduce joint inflammation, effusion and pain.

The tissues affected by manipulation are muscle, ligaments, tendons, joint capsules, articular surfaces, skin and fascia. These tissues are collectively term 'soft tissues'.

3

Manipulation and the repair processes

Probably one of the most common uses of manipulation is in aiding repair processes after musculo-skeletal injuries. By understanding the physiological mechanisms underlying tissue repair, treatment can be made more effective. This can help to reduce pain, accelerate healing and improve the mechanical and physiological properties of tissue.

PHYSIOLOGY OF CONNECTIVE TISSUE

The connective tissues refered to in this section are skin, fascia, ligaments, tendons, joint capsules and muscle fascia. Connective tissue is composed of the following:

- Extracellular components
  —Collagen, elastin and reticular fibres. These give the matrix its overall structure.
  —Water and glycosaminoglycans (GAGs). These provide lubrication and spacing between the collagen fibres.
- Cellular components
  —fibroblasts and chondrocytes which provide the 'materials' for making the matrix.

In tendons and ligaments, the cellular material makes up 20% of the total tissue volume, the extracellular matrix accounting for the remaining 80%. Water makes up 70% of the extracellular matrix, and the remaining 30% is composed of

9

solids. This high water content accounts for the tissue's viscous behaviour.[1,2]

Collagen and elastin

These fibres comprise the extracellular matrix and complement each other functionally. Collagen endows the tissue with strength and stiffness to resist mechanical force and deformation.[3,4] Elastin gives spring-like properties to the tissue, enabling it to recover from deformation.[4] Elastin and collagen fibres are intermingled and their ratio in connective tissue varies in different musculoskeletal structures. This ratio plays an important role in the overall mechanical properties of the tissue:[5] tissues rich in elastin have spring-like properties whereas tissues with high collagen content are generally stiffer.

Collagen, which is the main constituent of connective tissue, is synthesized by fibroblasts (Fig. 3.1).[6] Within the fibroblast, three chains of amino acids (procollagen) are synthesized and bound by intramolecular cross-links. Procollagen is then secreted by the fibroblasts to form extracellular tropocollagen molecules.[7] Once transported out of the cell, the collagen molecules are chemically bound to each other by intermolecular cross-links,[2] which 'glue' the molecular structure together to give the tissue its strength and stability under mechanical stress (Fig. 3.2). The collagen molecules aggregate in the extracellular matrix in a parallel arrangement to form microfibrils and then fibrils.[2] These aggregate further to form fibres, which are ultimately packed together to form the connective tissue suprastructures (tendon, ligaments, etc.). In newly formed collagen, the cross-links are relatively few and can easily be prised apart. In time, the cross-links mature and

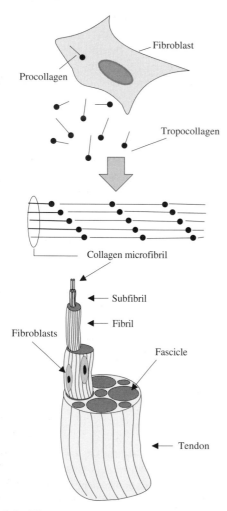

Figure 3.1 The stages of connective tissue formation.

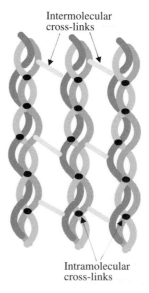

Figure 3.2 Inter- and intramolecular cross-links.

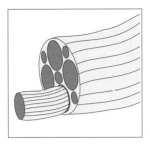

Fibre arrangement in tendon

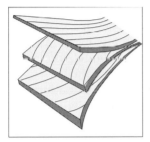

Fibre arrangement in ligaments

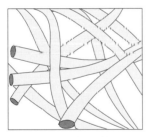

Fibre arrangement in skin

Figure 3.3   Collagen fibre arrangement in different connective tissues.

progressively become stronger.[8] During treatment of a new injury, excessive force should be avoided as it may damage the cross-links and lead to permanent mechanical weakness of the tissue.

The pattern of collagen deposition varies in different types of connective tissue (Fig. 3.3). It is an adaptive process related to the direction of forces imposed on the tissue.[9] In tendon, collagen fibres are organized in parallel arrangement; this gives the tendon stiffness and strength under unidirectional loads.[4] In ligaments, the organization of the fibres is looser, groups of fibres lying in different directions. This reflects the multidirectional forces that ligaments are subjected to, for example during complex movements of a joint such as flexion combined with rotation and shearing. The microorganization of collagen in the skin is arranged randomly. However, the skin is under constant tension, which means that the macroorganization of the skin follows a distinct pattern (Langer's lines).[10] The random pattern of collagen in the skin allows it to be stretched in all directions. When the skin is stretched in one direction, the collagen fibres transiently align parallel to the line of mechanical force. This type of alignment gives the skin great flexibility as well as high tensile strength.

Elastin has an arrangement similar to that of collagen in the extracellular matrix, and its deposition is also dependent on the mechanical stresses imposed on the tissue.[10]

Proteoglycans and water

Proteoglycans form the ground substance in which the collagen fibres are embedded. It is a viscous, gel-like substance that provides spacing and lubrication between the collagen microfibrils.[1,2,3] Where the fibrils intercept each other, this spacing prevents excessive cross-bridging, which would otherwise reduce the tissue's ability to deform (for example, during stretching). Proteoglycans are hydrophilic and draw water into the tissue. Their action can be likened to dipping a bud of cottonwool into water: the cotton bud will swell and expand as the water separates the cotton fibres. The hydrophilic properties of the proteoglycans produce a swelling pressure that is checked by the collagen fibres within the tissue matrix. In normal circumstances, the swelling pressure is in equilibrium with the tension created by the collagen fibres (Fig. 3.4). One could imagine what would happen were the fibres of the matrix to fail as can be seen following connective tissue injury; there would be little in the way of the tissue swelling.

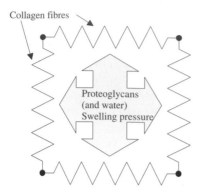

Figure 3.4 The swelling pressure produced by the proteoglycans is checked by the tensile properties of the collagen fibres.

Fibroblasts and chondrocytes

Fibroblasts and chondrocytes are the cellular components of connective tissue. They are the builders of connective tissue, synthesizing collagen, elastin and the precursors of proteoglycans. Fibroblasts are found in connective tissue such as ligaments, tendons, fascia and joint capsules. Chondrocytes are found in the collagen matrix of articular cartilage.

Their normal functioning depends on the extracellular environment and the deformation of the tissue which is brought about by movement. The fibroblasts and their daughter cells tend to align along the lines of stress in the tissue.[11] These stresses also activate intracellular messenger systems, stimulating the fibroblasts to modulate collagen,[1,2] elastin[11,12] and GAG synthesis.[1,2] This suggests that manipulation may affect cellular activity in the connective tissue matrix. The synthesis of the collagen matrix is counter-balanced by specialized enzymes which degrade and remove unneeded collagen, elastin and GAG.[1,2,10]

The internal cellular processes continue long after the cessation of the mechanical stimulus that initiated them. This implies that, although the manual event is transient, cellular processes may continue for some time after the treatment.

PHYSIOLOGICAL CHANGES IN TISSUES DURING INJURY, IMMOBILIZATION AND REMOBILIZATION

SOFT-TISSUE CHANGES FOLLOWING INJURY

Connective tissue changes

Injuries such as joint sprains will result in damage to the structure of the tissue. This damage is usually in the form of tears, which can be microscopic, affecting a limited number of collagen fibres, or large, affecting the whole tissue. In response to damage, the body initiates a repair process: inflammation (Fig. 3.5). The fact that inflammation is a positive process can be sometimes forgotten. The inflammatory response can be seen to have two major roles:

1. to protect the body from infection and clear tissue debris from the site of injury
2. in structural repair processes that take place at the site of damage.

Two types of cellular event are responsible for repair: one immunological, the other reparative. The immunological processes start immediately after injury. Cellular mechanisms are activated to prevent bacteria and other foreign materials from entering the wound and to clear the wound of tissue debris. In essence, these cells sweep clean the wound site. This activity is carried out primarily by macrophages and leucocytes.[14,15] The activity of these cells usually reaches a peak within the first 2 days after injury. In parallel to the immune response, a structural 'glueing together' of the wound is initiated. Immediately following injury, the wound ends are held together by a combination of a blood clot, collagen and local cells that actively adhere to each other. The collagen that is initially deposited forms a weak mesh made of reticular fibres, forming the scaffolding for the future deposition of collagen fibres.[16] This adhesion has little mechanical strength and can be easily disturbed by stretching. On about day 2, local and migrating fibroblasts begin to synthesize the

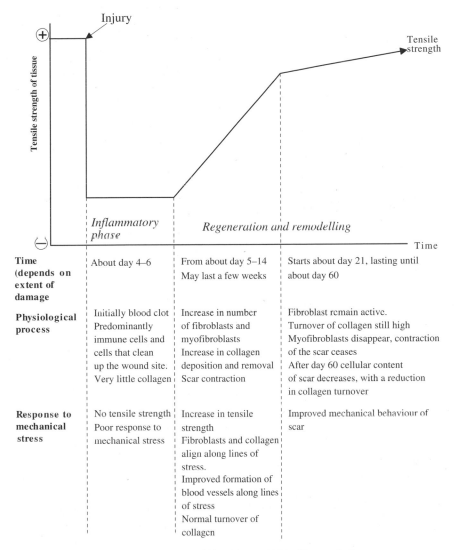

Figure 3.5 Stages in the repair process. (After Hunter 1994 with permission from the Chartered Society of Physiotherapy.[13])

collagen matrix needed to repair the wound.[14,17] The main increase in the deposition of collagen fibres (fibroplasia) starts on about the fifth day and reaches its peak on about day 14, continuing for perhaps 3–4 weeks.[18] During that time, there is an almost equal degradation and removal of collagen fibres. After the remodelling period, the cellular content of the scar gradually decreases. However, there still is a high turnover of collagen until about day 120. Thereafter, there is a gradual decrease in the number of fibroblasts and in

collagen turnover. This process may last up to a year after injury.[15] Throughout the repair and remodelling phases, there is a progressive increase in the tensile strength of the tissue (Fig. 3.5), which will determine the forces that can be used during manipulation. This will be discussed in Chapter 4.

In the early stages of repair, the cellular metabolic activity rises dramatically. To support this activity, new blood vessels regenerate at the site of repair. The *milieu* of these cells is highly dependent on the vascular delivery and removal of various substances.[19] It could be that, during these early stages, techniques that stimulate blood flow through the area could facilitate the transport of substances to and away from the repair site (see Ch. 5).

Repair in muscle

Muscle damage and repair are a common occurrence in physical activity such as exercise.[20–23] Skeletal muscle has a great capacity for regeneration, and this can occur without the formation of scar tissue. Immediately following trauma, there is damage and loss of the normal appearance of the muscle filaments and their surrounding cellular elements, with distension of the tissue space between the fibres by oedema.[24] Within a few hours, inflammatory cells appear in the area of damage. This process is similar to the inflammatory events seen in connective tissue. By the day 4–6, most of the cellular debris is cleared and a regeneration of muscle fibres can be seen. Activated satellite cells fuse to form myotubes, which progressively develop into muscle fibres. This regeneration process is very similar to that of normal myogenesis in the young. As the muscle fibres regenerate and increase in size, there is a concomitant decrease in the collagen content of the tissue. The regeneration process is usually completed by the third week.

Generally, muscle regeneration is quite rapid. For example, in the small muscles of the hand, this process can be completed in less than 7 days.[25] All but the most severe rupture will usually repair and regenerate without a significant increase in the content of connective tissue, i.e. scar tissue.[26] This potential for regeneration has been demonstrated in severe fractures, where there may be complete rupture and extensive damage to the muscle tissue.[24] For regeneration and restoration of normal function, it is essential that the blood and nerve supply to the muscle are not interrupted by the injury, and that tissue loss is not extensive. The importance of mechanical stress for normal repair and regeneration of muscle is discussed further in this chapter.

CHANGES WITH IMMOBILIZATION

Rigid immobilization as well as reduced range of movement will lead to adverse tissue changes, which may take place anywhere from cellular/matrix to gross tissue level (see Fig. 3.8 below):

Collagen matrix

With immobilization, there is an overall increase in the production and lysis of collagen. Without movement, the newly formed collagen is deposited in a random fashion, which reduces the overall tensile strength of the tissue (as the tensile strength of collagen is greater when the fibres are aligned along the lines of mechanical stress).

There is a decrease in GAG and water content of the matrix, allowing closer contact between the collagen fibrils and loss of lubrication.[27,28] This leads to the formation of abnormal points of cross-linking between the fibres, restricting normal interfibril gliding.[28] It is believed that the mechanism behind the loss of extensibility results not from the volume of collagen deposited but from the area in which it is deposited.[29] A dramatic reduction in the tissue's overall mobility may occur from the formation of abnormal cross-links at strategic points where the gliding fibrils come into close contact (Fig. 3.6).[27,29]

Ligaments

In immobilized joints, ligaments lose strength and stiffness and their insertion points are weakened (Fig. 3.7).[30,31] Prolonged immobilization results in reduced collagen content and atrophy of the ligaments.[32,33]

It should be noted that stiffness is not a negative property of connective tissue as it provides support and strength to areas of the body that are under high tensile stresses; for example, the plantar ligaments of the foot need to be fairly stiff to prevent the arch of the foot collapsing.

Tendons

Immobilized tendons atrophy, with degradation

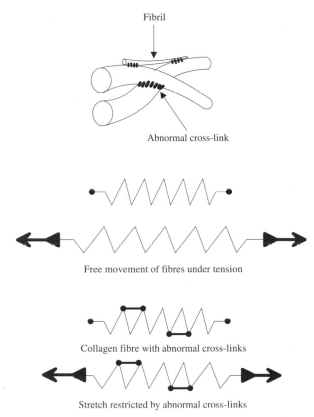

Figure 3.6 Abnormal cross-links and the deposition of newly synthesized fibrils may reduce the overall extendibility of the tissue.

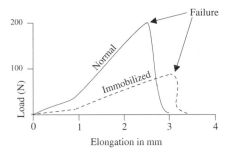

Figure 3.7 Changes in the mechanical strength of ligaments following immobilization. After Amiel et al[31] with permission)

of their mechanical properties. This is often accompanied by extensive obliteration of the space between the tendon and its sheath as a result of adhesions. This severely impedes the gliding action of the tendon within its sheath,

reducing the joint's overall range of movement.[34] The regeneration of the vascular supply to the healing tendon is also affected by immobilization, resulting in poor, random growth of blood vessels.

Muscle

Muscle is the main tissue to undergo shortening and is often the cause of restriction of the range of movement in immobilized joints. Such changes in length are due to adaptive sarcomere and connective tissue changes.[35] It has been demonstrated that in muscle immobilized in its shortened length, there is a reduction in the number of sarcomeres (40% within a few days) but with an increase in their length. This is accompanied by shortening and proliferation of the muscle's connective tissue elements (epimysium, perimysium and endomysium).[1,24] Without movement or muscle contraction, there may be excessive oedema and stasis in the tissue spaces.[24] Some of the changes in innervated and denervated immobilized muscle are very similar, suggesting that the structural changes are largely a result of the absence of mechanical stress on muscle tissue.[35]

It has been proposed that similar structural changes in muscles occur in patients with long-term spasticity. In this state, the muscle is continuously being used or held in a shortened length, which leads to a reduction in the number of sarcomeres and connective tissue elements. Such changes account for some of the stiffness and reduced extendibility of muscle during passive stretching.[35]

Peri- and intra-articular tissues

The capsule, ligaments and synovial membrane progressively atrophy during immobilization. Adhesion and abnormal cross-links result in contracture formation and reduced overall movement of the joint. The synovial tissue of immobilized joints seems to be the most sensitive to the effects of immobilization and undergoes fibrofatty changes. The resultant fibrofatty tissue proliferates into all the articular soft tissues, for example in the knee, into the cruciate ligament and the undersurface of the quadriceps tendon. With the passage of time, fibrofatty changes will proliferate to cover the non-articulating area of cartilage, with the subsequent formation of adhesions between the two surfaces as the fibrofatty tissue matures. The proliferation of fibrofatty tissue and adhesion formation has been shown to occur as early as 15 days after immobilization, becoming well established after 30 days.[30,36] These changes have been shown to occur in experimental animals as well as in human intervertebral and knee joints.[30,35,37,38] In the knee, similar but less extensive changes have been observed in subjects with damage to the anterior cruciate ligament. Adhesion formation and fibrosis have been found between the patellar fat pad and the synovium adjacent to the damaged ligament.[38]

Immobilization also affects the articular cartilage. The chondrocytes in the articular cartilage are totally dependent on synovial fluid for their nutrition. As the synovial membrane progressively atrophies, there may be a decrease in nutrition and gradual destruction of the articular cartilage.

ADHESIONS, CONTRACTION, CONTRACTURES, CROSS-LINKS AND SCAR TISSUE

Adhesions

Adhesions are abnormal deposits of connective tissue between two gliding surfaces, such as tendons and their sheath or capsular fold, as in adhesive capsulitis.[28] Once matured, these abnormal connections can be stronger than the tissue to which they adhere. For example, stretching intra-articular adhesions can avulse the cartilage to which they adhere rather than tear the ligaments themselves. Thus, in such a situation, forceful manipulation may damage the parent tissue without affecting the adhesion. In some conditions, providing movement is not impaired, the adhesions will disappear in time. This is probably due to the remodelling processes to which the adhesions together with other

connective tissues, are subjected.[39] For example, the severe loss of movement in frozen shoulder may (on occasions) resolve without any attempt by the patient to exercise or seek treatment. Low-level or very 'young' adhesions can probably be broken down by stretching.

Contraction

After injury, one usually experiences a tightening of the scar, which is brought about by contraction of the myofibroblasts pulling the free ends of the wound towards each other.[17,19,40–42] The myofibroblast is a cross between fibroblast and myocyte and has contractile abilities (having, like muscle cells, contractile proteins). Articulating joints within their full range of movement can reduce excessive contraction formation.[42]

Contractures

The term 'contracture' is usually used to indicate a loss of joint range of movement as a result of connective tissue and muscle shortening. Underlying contracture formation are adhesions or excessive cross-links.[43] Depending on their extent, contractures can be reduced by stretching or movement.[44]

Cross-links

Cross-links, as described above, are the chemical bonds within and between the collagen molecules. Abnormal cross-linking can reduce the extendibility of the tissue. Cross-links are discussed in more detail throughout this chapter.

Scar tissue

Scar tissue results from the overall cellular and matrix changes in a tissue that take place following damage. Many of the processes described above are seen in the formation of scar tissue.

RESTORING HOMEOSTASIS BY MOVEMENT

Exercise or manipulation can normalize connective tissue homeostasis following injury (Fig. 3.8). There is a strong body of evidence to support the view that periodic, moderate stress is essential for tissue nutrition healing and viability.[21] The mode of manipulation is very important to the outcome of the repair (modes of tissue loading are discussed later). For example, tensile forces will increase aggregation of collagen, resulting in thicker and denser tissue, thus improving the tissue's stiffness and strength. Compression, in contrast, has the opposite effect, resulting in thinner and mechanically low-quality tissue.[45] The ultrastructure of the tissue will also depend on the type of technique used. For example, continuous stretching will result in structurally longer tissue even in the presence of scar contraction.[15,46]

Although, in many of the following studies, continuous passive motion was used, it has been shown that even periodic passive motion can

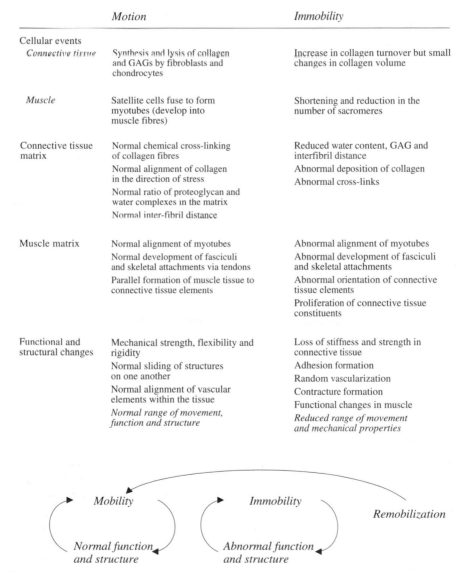

	Motion	*Immobility*
Cellular events		
Connective tissue	Synthesis and lysis of collagen and GAGs by fibroblasts and chondrocytes	Increase in collagen turnover but small changes in collagen volume
Muscle	Satellite cells fuse to form myotubes (develop into muscle fibres)	Shortening and reduction in the number of sacromeres
Connective tissue matrix	Normal chemical cross-linking of collagen fibres Normal alignment of collagen in the direction of stress Normal ratio of proteoglycan and water complexes in the matrix Normal inter-fibril distance	Reduced water content, GAG and interfibril distance Abnormal deposition of collagen Abnormal cross-links
Muscle matrix	Normal alignment of myotubes Normal development of fasciculi and skeletal attachments via tendons Parallel formation of muscle tissue to connective tissue elements	Abnormal alignment of myotubes Abnormal development of fasciculi and skeletal attachments Abnormal orientation of connective tissue elements Proliferation of connective tissue constituents
Functional and structural changes	Mechanical strength, flexibility and rigidity Normal sliding of structures on one another Normal alignment of vascular elements within the tissue *Normal range of movement, function and structure*	Loss of stiffness and strength in connective tissue Adhesion formation Random vascularization Contracture formation Functional changes in muscle *Reduced range of movement and mechanical properties*

Figure 3.8   Effects of motion, immobilization and remobilization on connective tissue and muscle homeostasis, function and structure.

stimulate the healing processes and improve the mechanical properties of the tissue.[47,48]

Connective tissue matrix

Movement encourages the normal turnover of collagen and its alignment along the lines of stress. This provides the tissue with better tensile properties. Movement improves the balance of GAGs and water content within the tissue which help maintain the inter-fibril distance and lubrication (Fig. 3.8). This reduces the potential for abnormal cross-links formation and adhesion. In avascular structures, such as cartilage, ligaments and tendons, periodic stress provides a pumping effect for the flow of interstitial fluid. This may support the increased metabolic needs of the tissue during inflammation and repair.[19,21]

Joints

Movement produces pressure fluctuations within the joint cavity that are important for the formation and removal of synovial fluid.[27] Movement also encourages the smearing of synovial fluid onto the articular surface. The synovial fluid is an important nutritional route for the chondrocytes as the articular cartilage has no blood supply.[49] Cyclical stress brought about by movement stimulates the metabolic activity of chondrocytes, resulting in proteoglycan and collagen synthesis.[50] The viability and repair of the articular cartilage depends on these processes. In mobilized joints, it has been shown that small defects in the articular surfaces can heal by hyaline cartilage, rather than fibro-cartilage, as found in immobilized animals.[51,52] Intra-articular adhesions formed during immobilization were shown to be reduced by the animal's return to free movement.[36]

Ligaments

Passive motion has been shown to stimulate various aspects of healing in ligaments. If a knee is mobilized early, the ligaments show higher strength and stiffness compared with immobilized ligaments (providing that the joint movements are not excessive and scar formation is not disturbed).[53] Similarly, the strength of healing ligaments has been shown to be superior in animals allowed to exercise.[33]

Muscle

As with other tissues in the body, muscle regeneration is dependent on longitudinal mechanical tension, provided by either passive stretching or muscle contraction. Longitudinal tension promotes the normal parallel alignment of the myotubes to the lines of stress,[24,26] and is required for the restoration of the connective tissue component of the regeneration muscle.[24] Without the development of internal tendons, fasciculi and adequate well-defined skeletal attachments, muscle function will not be restored, even where muscle fibre regeneration has taken place.[26] During remobilization of muscle, the number and size of the sarcomeres generally return to preimmobilization levels.[35] Animal studies show that passive muscle stretching leads to increased muscle length, hypertrophy and increased capillary density.[54] In human subjects with osteoarthritis of the hip, passive (transverse) muscle stretching has been shown significantly to increase the range of movement as well as the cross-sectional area of muscle fibres and their glycogen content (decreased muscle mobility leading to muscle atrophy and reduced glycogen content).[54]

Tissue culture experiments highlight the importance of both stress and motion to healing. Passive stretching of muscle activates intracellular mechanisms that result in hypertrophy (increase in cell size) of the muscle cell.[55] Smooth muscle cells that are cyclically stretched demonstrate increased synthesis of proline, a major constituent of collagen. Agitation of the culture medium does not increase the cellular metabolism to the same extent. This suggests that the increase seen with intermittent stretching is not due to pumping of nutrients by movement but is a cellular response to changes in the mechanical environment.[56] Studies using skeletal tissue culture have shown that muscle cells incubated under constant tension synthesize protein at 22%

of the rate observed in vivo, whereas passive intermittent stretching resulted in a level of 38% of that found in vivo.[57] This suggests that the changing patterns of mechanical stress are more potent than static events at stimulating such cellular events. The clinical implication may be that treatment of muscle injury should follow similar mechanical patterns, i.e. rhythmic cyclical stretches or muscle contractions.

The structural changes seen in muscle tissue during immobilization can be minimized by early mobilization. Passive and active movement will encourage parallel formation of muscle tissue with its connective tissue elements, and will help to reduce oedema and stasis. Active techniques will stimulate muscle fibre regeneration, a normal ratio of muscle to connective tissue elements, and the development of neuromuscular connections.

Tendons

Healing tendons that undergo mobilization have a higher tensile strength and rupture less often than immobilized tendons.[58] Early mobilization of an injured tendon reduces the proliferation of fibrotic tissue and reduces the formation of adhesions between the tendon and its sheath.[59,60] Animal experiments have shown that tendons undergoing early mobilization are stronger than immobilized tendons. At 12 weeks post-operation, the angular rotation of the tendon of the immobilized group was 19% of the full range of movement. Mobilization delayed until after 3 weeks post-operation produced an angular rotation of 67%, while the early mobilized group showed an angular rotation of 95% of the full range of movement.[58] In the early mobilization group, passive motion was initiated within 5 days of the operation. The total DNA and cellularity content of mobilized tendons at the repair site were significantly higher than was found in immobilized tendons,[61] increased DNA and cellularity signifying an acceleration in tendon repair and maturation.

Motion also stimulated the reorientation and revascularization of the blood vessels at the site of healing in a more normal pattern; immobiliza-

tion produces a random vascular regeneration pattern.

An indication to manual therapists of the rate and time needed to effect such changes has been given in studies on the rate of tendon healing in animals.[62] Two groups of animals were given 60 cycles of flexion and extension over two periods of time: 5 minutes and 60 minutes. Both groups were manually articulated on a daily basis. The 5 minutes group displayed better healing and strength of the tendon than did the 60 minute group. It was suggested that the healing process was facilitated by a higher frequency of articulation. In a study of adhesive capsulitis, oscillatory-type articulation for 3–6 minutes per session was shown significantly to increase the range of joint movement and to be more effective than sustained stretches.[39] The length of manipulation in this study falls well within the practical limitations of a manual treatment. As the healing process in most connective tissue is generally of a similar nature, the therapeutic implications of these studies could be loosely applied to other connective tissues.

Skin

Wound healing in skin has also been shown to be affected by mechanical stimuli, mechanically stressed scars being much stronger and stiffer than unstressed scars. The mechanical properties of a scar closely resemble those of normal skin, the collagen fibres developing in a biaxial orientation. The cosmetic appearance of a scar healed under mechanical loading is greatly superior to that of unstressed scar.[40,63,64]

MOVEMENT: THE BLUEPRINT FOR NORMAL FUNCTIONAL AND STRUCTURAL PROPERTIES OF TISSUE

Studies of tissue repair, immobility and remobilization all demonstrate the importance of movement for normal repair processes and tissue health. Movement provides direction to the deposition of collagen, maintains a balance between the connective tissue constituents, encourages normal vascular regeneration and reduces the formation of excessive cross-links and adhesions.

Movement is the blueprint for normal structural and functional properties of muscle and connective tissues. Tissues that have healed under movement and mechanical stress will have properties matching the mechanical requirements of daily physical activities. Tissues that have healed while immobile, or under reduced or abnormal movement, may fail to meet the imposed structural and functional demands of daily activities (Fig. 3.9).

MANIPULATION IN THE DIFFERENT PHASES OF REPAIR

The cellular sequence during repair will pro-

foundly influence the choice of techniques used throughout the healing process. In the early stages, the tissue has little mechanical strength and any stretching will therefore disturb and separate the wound ends. At this point, the aim of manipulation is to support the metabolic needs of the inflammatory cells by facilitating blood and lymph flow through the tissue. Rhythmic non-painful techniques can be used here (see Ch. 5). Following the inflammatory phase, the aim of manipulation is to direct the repair and remodelling process. The remodelling process is more readily affected when the scar is young (Fig. 3.10),[11] owing to three main factors:

1. As the scar matures, the turnover of the matrix constituents is diminished, reducing the potential for remodelling.

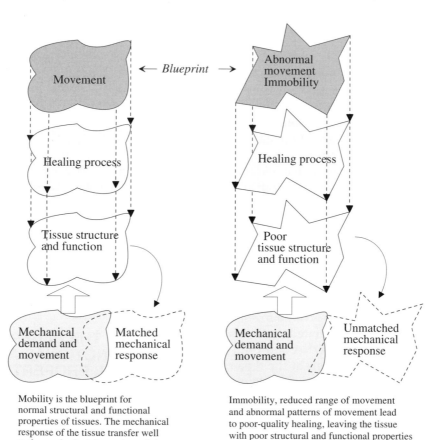

Mobility is the blueprint for normal structural and functional properties of tissues. The mechanical response of the tissue transfer well to the mechanical demands made by movement

Immobility, reduced range of movement and abnormal patterns of movement lead to poor-quality healing, leaving the tissue with poor structural and functional properties

Figure 3.9 The blueprint for healing tissue with or without mobility.

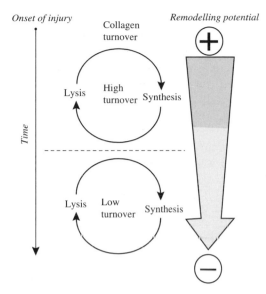

Figure 3.10 The potential for remodelling decreases as scar tissue matures.

2. In mature scar, the bonding between the collagen molecules is stronger and therefore less easily disrupted by stretching.[65]

3. Adhesions and excessive cross-links may be present in more mature scar tissue, especially when movement has not been introduced during the early stages of repair.

This highlights the need to introduce treatment soon after injury. The aim at this stage is to provide a movement background for the re-modelling process; cyclical movement can be used. In time, as the tissue regains its tensile strength, the force of manipulation and the range of movement can progressively be increased (see Ch. 4). Treatment is eventually superseded by the patient's return to daily activities, which will provide the long-term stimulus needed for the remodelling process.

4

The biomechanical response

Clinically, manipulation is often used to re-establish the structural and functional properties of tissue, such as by elongating shortened tissue, and improving flexibility and strength.

Tissues will respond to different types of manipulation. Some techniques will be effective in producing a change, whereas others will fail to alter the structural and functional properties of the tissue. This chapter examines how different modes of manipulation can be made more effective in producing the intended change.

MODES OF TISSUE LOADING

The mode by which a tissue is loaded will determine its eventual structural changes. Most manual techniques can be categorized according to the changes they impose on tissues and joints. These are called the modes of loading (Fig. 4.1):[2]

- tension loading
- compression loading
- rotation loading
- bending loading
- shearing loading
- combined loading.

Tension loading

This is also termed traction, elongation, longitudinal stretching and extension. Tissues elongate under tensile loading, which is therefore used to lengthen shortened tissues. During repair and

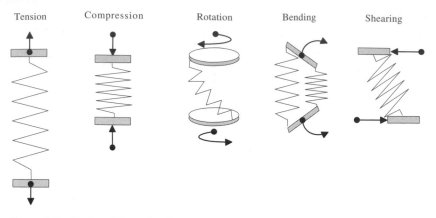

Figure 4.1 Modes of tissue loading.

remodelling, tensile forces cause an increase in the aggregation of collagen, resulting in thicker and denser tissue, thus improving the tissue's stiffness and strength. Sustained compression, in contrast, has the opposite effect, resulting in thinner and mechanically poorer-quality tissue.[4–5]

Tension will minimally affect fluid flow. This principle can be demonstrated using a wet mop as an analogy: if the mop is forcefully pulled at its two ends, there is elongation of the fibres but little loss of water.

Compression loading

Under compressive loads, the tissue will shorten and widen, increasing the pressure within the tissue and affecting fluid flow. Compression is therefore a very useful pump-like technique to facilitate the flow of fluid. Compression, however, will be ineffective as a stretching technique. Using the wet mop analogy, if a wet mop is squeezed, there is an outflow of fluids without elongation of the mop's fibres.

In a direct soft-tissue technique applied to the muscle, both fibre length and fluid flow may be affected by the combination of tissue compression and elongation.

Rotation loading

Rotation has a complex mechanical effect on tissue, being a combination of compression of the whole structure, and a progressive elongation of the fibres furthest away from the axis of rotation (think of wringing a wet mop). Rotation mode relates largely to articulation techniques rather than soft-tissue techniques, i.e. joints can be rotated but muscle cannot be twisted by massage.

Bending loading

Bending is expressed anatomically as flexion, extension or side-bending. The bending form of loading subjects the tissue to a combination of tension and compression (tension on the convex and compression on the concave side). Bending can be used as a tension technique to elongate shortened tissue and for stimulating flow, such as in joint articulation.

Shearing loading

Shearing is mainly used in joint articulation. As with rotation, it will produce a complex pattern of compression and elongation of fibres.

Combined loading

Combined loading is the simultaneous application of any number of loading modes, for example, side-bending combined with rotation. With the addition of each successive mode, there is a cumulative tension effect on the tissue. This may be more effective than stretching in only one mode, for example, side-bending combined with traction is a stronger form of stretching than is side-bending or traction alone.

Tension and compression underlie all of the different modes of loading. It can be argued that, in essence, any form of manipulation is either in tension, compression or a combination of these modes. Tension is important in conditions where tissues need to be elongated, whereas compression is more useful in conditions where fluid flow needs to be affected. The effects of tension on tissue biomechanics are discussed in this chapter, whilst the effect of compression on fluid dynamics is discussed in more detail in Chapter 5.

VISCOELASTICITY

The mechanical behaviour of soft tissues is related to the overall property of connective tissue called *viscoelasticity*.[1,2,4,66,67] As its name implies, viscoelasticity is a function of a composite, a biological material that contains a combination of stiff and elastic fibres embedded in a gel medium. This gives the tissue the mechanical properties of its individual components as well as a unique behaviour that does not reside in either constituent. Elasticity is the spring-like element within the tissue.[4] Viscous properties are the dampening and lubricating elements. Normally, there is a balance between elasticity and viscosity. Excessive elasticity would mean that with any movement our body would excessively and uncontrollably vibrate and bounce on the ground, like a rubber ball. Such a system would need extensive muscle activity to stabilize the body. Similarly, excessive dampening forces would also require increased muscular activity to overcome these forces and to compensate for the loss of spring and pendular mechanisms in the body.[68]

The different mechanical properties of collagen can be depicted by a spring, for the elastic component, and a piston, for the viscous component (Fig. 4.2). The upper and lower parts of the piston chamber are interconnected to allow flow

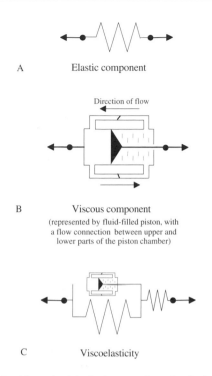

A   Elastic component

Direction of flow

B   Viscous component
(represented by fluid-filled piston, with a flow connection between upper and lower parts of the piston chamber)

C   Viscoelasticity

Figure 4.2   Viscoelasticity is the overall mechanical property of connective tissue.

between the two chambers. The diameter of the interconnection will determine the resistance to flow. A piston in parallel with a spring element is well suited to represent the viscous changes occurring over time. A piston unit without a spring unit in parallel can represent the plastic component of collagen. These various components, put together in parallel and in series, represent the combined mechanical properties of soft tissue.[69]

THE STRESS–STRAIN CURVE

When a tissue is stretched, it will display a characteristic stress–strain curve with different structural changes occurring at each region of the curve.[1,2] The stress–strain curve has three distinct regions (Fig. 4.3):

- toe region
- elastic region (also called linear range)
- plastic region.

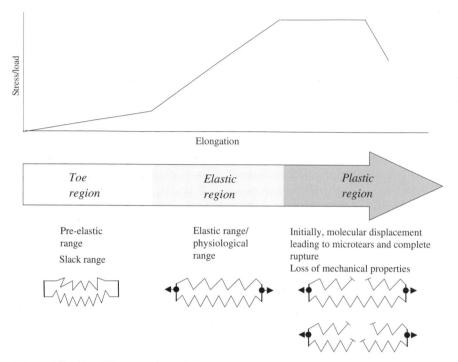

Figure 4.3 The different regions of the stress-strain curve.

TOE REGION

The initial elongation of the tissue reflects the straightening and flattening of the wavy configuration of the tissue (Fig. 4.4).[70] The toe regions account for 1.5–4% of the total tissue length.[2] In this region, there is no true elastic elongation of the tissue: once the stretch is removed, the tissue will return to its original wavy configuration. Some tissues have longer toe regions depending on the waviness of the collagen pattern. For

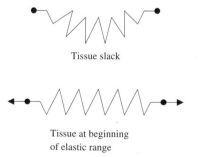

Figure 4.4 In the toe region, there is no true elongation of the collagen fibres.

example, in tendons, the collagen lies in an almost parallel pattern and the toe region is therefore very small, whereas ligaments that have some wavy structure have a longer toe region. In manual therapy, this area is often referred to as 'slack', hence use of the term 'to take out the slack' before stretching.

In tendons, the stress needed to flatten the toe region was found to be equal to maximal contraction of the muscle.[71] This implies that during passive muscle stretching most of the elongation will take place in the muscle belly rather than its tendon.

ELASTIC REGION

The second region of the curve is the elastic region, in which the tissue displays spring-like properties, and length changes in the tissue are directly proportional to the applied forces. This linear relationship is the hallmark of elastic structures (Fig. 4.5). The overall elasticity of the tissue is determined by the ratio of elastin to collagen.

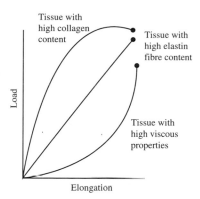

Figure 4.5 The stress–strain curve of different connective tissues.

For example, the ligamentum nuci and liga-mentum flavum have a high elastin content (70%) and are therefore very elastic.[4,67] Elastic tissue with its high elastin content, has a more horizontal stress–strain curve, whereas if the tissue is rich in collagen, it will be stiffer, showing a more vertical stress–strain curve.

The elastic region accounts for tissue elonga-tion of 2–5%.[2] During stretching in this region,

the fibres straighten out, begin to elongate and become progressively stiffer. The more elastic a tissue is, the longer will be the elastic region without failure of the collagen fibres. Tissues with a high collagen content, for example tendons, have shorter toe and elastic regions.

Depending on the type of tissue, most physio-logical movement occurs within the toe and end-elastic ranges. In tendons, the stress needed to flatten the toe region has been found to be equal to maximal contraction of the muscle.[71] In comparison, skin is more elastic, and most of its physiological movement occurs throughout the elastic range without any failure.[8]

Creep deformation

If, during stretching in the elastic range, the tissue is held at a constant length, there will be a slow elongation of the tissue. This elongation is a *transient* biomechanical phenomenon called 'creep deformation' (Fig. 4.6). When unloaded, the tissue will not return immediately to its

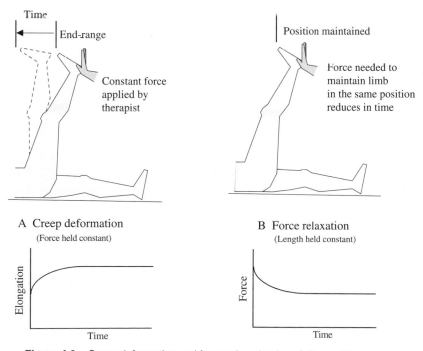

Figure 4.6 Creep deformation and force relaxation in soft tissue. These are biomechanical responses related to viscoelasticity and are not neurologically mediated.

original prestretched length. This transient imperfect recovery is believed to be due to the viscous or fluid-like property of collagen.[4,72] During loading, there is a slow seeping of fluids out of the tissue matrix, and vice versa, when the tissue is unloaded: there is a slow absorption of fluid into the tissue.[21]

When a tissue is repeatedly stretched, there is an increment of elongation with each successive cycle, a phenomenon also associated with creep deformation. This increment of elongation decreases with each cycle until a steady state is reached at which the tissue will not elongate any further. At this length, the tissue is said to be 'preconditioned'. It has been shown that, during cyclical stretching of the muscle–tendon unit, some 80% of elongation will take place in the first four cycles of stretching.[73]

Creep deformation is time dependent, i.e. tissue elongation is related to the rate at which it is being stretched. Therefore, creep changes tend to occur during slow-rather than high-velocity stretching.

Force relaxation

If, during stretching, the tissue is held at a set length, there is a progressive reduction in the force needed to maintain that length. This phenomenon is called 'force relaxation' (Fig. 4.6).[1,2] For example, in the anterior longitudinal ligament, the force needed to maintain the ligament at a constant length is almost halved within the first minute.[4]

The rate at which the force is applied will also affect the resulting relaxation of the tissue. The more rapid the force, the shorter the time it takes the tissue to relax.[4,73] However, it is dangerous to rely on this property to stretch tissues as high-velocity (fast) stretching may exceed the tissue's ability to undergo creep changes (which, it should be remembered, are time dependent)[4] and may result in microtears in the stretched tissue. This may be further compounded during stretching of damaged tissue that has a lower tensile strength.

Creep deformation and force relaxation are palpable properties of soft tissues. They can be demonstrated by slowly stretching a finger into extension until there is a barrier to the movement, and maintaining this position for a few seconds. After a while, there will be a sensation of 'give' and the joint will move into further extension. This process can be repeated a few times with successive stretches of the tissue up to the next barrier/length. What is sensed are creep deformation and stress relaxation of the antagonist tissues. In practice, providing the patient is fully relaxed and there is no underlying neurological muscle tone, most relaxation phenomena of stretched tissue are related to biomechanical rather than neurological changes (see Section 2).

Hysteresis

During stretching, there is a discrepancy between the mechanical energy used to stretch the tissue and the energy required to return the tissue to its original shape (the latter being called the relaxation phase). The relaxation phase is somewhat longer than the stretching phase (Fig. 4.7), partly due to the dissipation of mechanical energy as heat during the stretching phase. This means that not all the energy is conserved as elastic strain energy, and there is therefore less mechanical energy available for the recoil (relaxation phase). This discrepancy is also due to the rate of fluid flow in the tissue. The rate for outflow is faster than for flow back into the tissue.[4,73]

PLASTIC RANGE

As stretching approaches the end of the elastic range, there is progressive failure and microscopic tearing of the collagen fibres.[2,16] This is

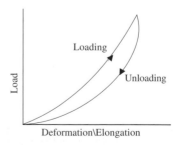

Figure 4.7 Hysteresis loop.

different from creep deformation that is associated with fluid flow. This region of the stress–strain curve is called the plastic region. Once stretching reaches the plastic region, the mechanical changes in the tissue are irreversible, so that even if the load is removed, the tissue will not return to its original length (Fig. 4.8) and will have lost some of its tensile strength. Further stretching within the plastic range will lead to a progressive increase in the number of fibres failing, until there is a complete rupture of the tissue. The point of rupture is represented at the abrupt end of the stress–strain curve (see Fig. 4.3 above). Following plastic changes, the return of the tissue to normal length and tensile strength is through inflammation and repair.

Collagen fibres have different lengths, thickness and directions. The shorter, thicker fibres will become maximally stretched or loaded before the longer, thinner ones. The fibres that are first to be fully stretched will also be the fibres that will be the first to tear.[16] Even in the early stages of the elastic range there may be microscopic failure of the collagen fibres.[71] This begins at about 3% of the tissue's resting length, and at about 6–10% (although this may vary between different tissues) there is complete rupture of the tissue.[2,74,75] For example, complete rupture of the anterior cruciate ligament occurs at about 7 mm of elongation, with microfailure occurring at lower strains.[2] Some studies put the safe stretching zone as being the toe region, i.e. about 1% to a maximum of 3%.[71,75] In practical terms, these percentages mean very little in a clinical situation where several structures, each with its own individual stress–strain curve, are stretched simultaneously. Furthermore, there is no way of knowing whether one is stretching to 2%, 4%, etc. The percentage length change is discussed simply to highlight the fact that, when stretching tendons, ligaments or joint capsules, one should not expect large visual changes: any length change will be in millimetres rather than centimetres.

MANUAL STRETCHING

Manual stretching can be divided into passive and active stretching. In passive stretching, the patient is fully relaxed while being manually stretched, whereas in active stretching, the patient's own muscle contraction provides the force needed to stretch the muscle.

PASSIVE STRETCHING

There are several variables that determine the safety, efficacy and level of discomfort during stretching; these will be discussed below.

Rate of stretching

Stretching should be performed slowly rather than rapidly, allowing the tissue to undergo viscous changes. In animal tendons, a low-load sustained stretching has been shown to be more effective at producing residual elongation than a high-load brief stretch.[69] In the human knee, it has similarly been shown that low-load sustained stretching is more effective than brief, high-load stretching in treating flexion deformities.[76]

Rapid stretching may exceed the tissue's ability to undergo viscous changes, resulting in further trauma and tearing. Indeed, most injuries occur during high-velocity activity. This is even more important when stretching a damaged tissue that has lost some of its mechanical strength. Rapid stretching will lead to a vicious cycle of damage and low-quality repair, or even to chronic inflammation.

In some instances where healing with adhesion has taken place, high-velocity stretching has been recommended to tear the adhesions.[77] This should be done with extreme caution so as not to

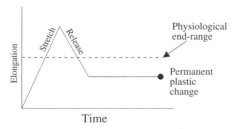

Figure 4.8 Plasticity can be demonstrated by stretching a tissue beyond its physiological end-range. When released, there is a permanent elongation of the fibres.

retraumatize the healed tissue. As described in Chapter 3, it should be noted that adhesions can be stronger than the tissue to which they are attached, so the need to introduce high-velocity stretching should be carefully considered. High-velocity stretching can possibly be used where adhesions are minimal or have not matured.

Soft tissues become stiffer at increasing rates (speed) of stretching (Fig. 4.9).[78] During rapid stretching, the tissue has elastic, spring-like behaviour. Only during slow or static stretching will there be effective elongation in the tissue. Therefore, in high velocity stretching there will be more of a 'kick back' from the stretched tissue as the stiffer it will feel.[4,73] Ideally, stretching should be slow and gradual. For this reason the ballistic type of stretching is currently out of vogue in sports.

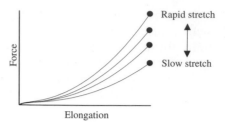

Figure 4.9   Progressively rapid stretching results in a stiffer and more elastic mechanical response.

Force of loading

The use of force should be considered carefully in relation to the different phases of tissue repair (Fig. 4.10).[13] Manipulation will affect the different repair phases contributing to the improvement in the tissue's mechanical properties and length.

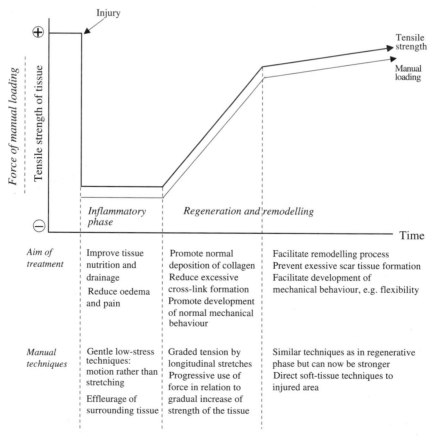

Figure 4.10   Tensile strength of soft tissue following injury. Manual considerations during the different healing phases. (After Hunter 1994 with permission from the Chartered Society of Physiotherapy.[13])

During the inflammatory phase, the tissue has a low tensile strength and can easily be disturbed by heavy-handed manipulation. Following injury, some fibres are torn and the mechanical integrity of the tissue rests on fewer intact fibres. At this stage of repair, stretching should be minimal or avoided altogether; movement may be more appropriate to facilitate the resolution of the inflammatory phase. The use of movement is discussed in more detail in Chapter 5. During the regenerative and remodelling phases, the tissue progressively regains its tensile strength and the manual forces can be increased in a graded manner. To gauge the force and amplitude of stretching, the therapist has to rely on the levels of tension created in the tissues and the discomfort it causes. My personal guidelines on amplitude and force often rely on the amount of pain and discomfort that the stretch is inflicting. A 'pleasant' stretching sensation that feels 'therapeutic' is usually acceptable, whereas I avoid stretching that inflicts sharp, burning or severe pain. The level of damage also has to be assessed before stretching commences. How to assess this in a tissue is beyond the scope of this book, but general consideration such as the mode of injury, clinical signs and symptoms can help to build up an understanding of the nature of injury. One important guideline is how 'fresh' the injury is. Stretching should be avoided if the injury is acute or recent with an onset of up to 2 weeks.

A further consideration is that, in injury, several tissues may be damaged simultaneously. As each has its own rate of healing, there may be superimposition of the different phases, for example, those of highly vascularized tissue (such as muscle) with its rapid healing rate being superimposed on those of a less vascularized tissue (such as ligament), with its slower healing rate. Stretching may have to be postponed until the inflammatory phase has been completed in all the tissues.

Duration of stretch

There are some difficulties in defining how long a tissue should be held in stretch to undergo length changes. Different variables, such as the force used, the diameter and length of the tissue, the level of tissue damage, and inflammation and scar formation, will affect this duration. The recommended time for stretching a muscle tendon unit (to a length just short of pain) is anywhere from 6 to 60 seconds.[73] In the hamstrings of normal individuals, it has been found that a single daily episode of stretching for 30 seconds is significantly more effective than that for 15 seconds. However, there are no significant differences between stretches lasting 30 and 60 seconds,[79] implying that the duration of stretch is most effective at about 30 seconds. However, because of structural and morphological diversity, it is almost impossible to predict the duration of stretching for each tissue. Decisions on the level of force and duration of stretch are ultimately perceived by palpation, feeling for a change in length of the tissue. The ability to detect such changes can improve with practice.

Mode of loading

Connective tissue and muscle–tendon units have complex anatomical organizations, with fibres running at different angles and anchoring to multiple insertion and origin points. Different modes of loading can be used to stretch these different fibres (Fig. 4.11).

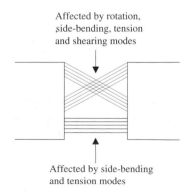

Figure 4.11 Various modes of manual loading will affect different fibres of the tissue.

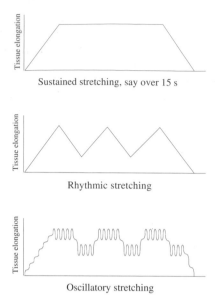

Figure 4.12 Different forms of stretching.

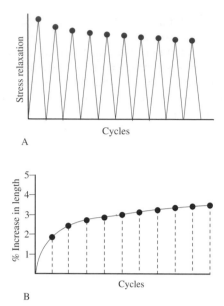

Figure 4.13 The effect of cyclic stretches on the muscle–tendon unit. (A) Stress relaxation curve of a muscle–tendon unit repeatedly stretched to 10% beyond its resting length. Most relaxation took place in the first four stretches. The overall relaxation was 16.6%. (B) Creep deformation of the muscle–tendon unit with repeated stretching to the same tension. Eighty per cent of the length increase occurred during the first four stretches. (After Taylor et al 1990 with permission.[73])

Cyclical stretching

Continuous and static stretching can be uncomfortable to the patient. For example, if you stretch your own finger into full extension and hold it for 15 seconds pain will develop very rapidly in the stretched tissues. Clinically, this situation may be compounded during stretches of damaged painful tissues. Cyclical, rhythmic stretching of tissues offers an alternative to continuous stretching as it does not inflict the same level of pain and discomfort (Fig. 4.12). This type of stretching is, in some ways, more natural as it involves periods of tissue stress and destress. A destressing period is needed to allow the tissue (and the patient) to relax from the discomfort of stretching. Movement during stretching may also have a neurological influence on the perception of pain (see Ch. 12).

In cyclical stretching, the forces used in each loading cycle may be relatively small but there is a cumulative effect on the tissue.[20] When the muscle–tendon unit is cyclically stretched to a fixed tension and a fixed length, there is an increment of elongation (creep) and stress relaxation with each stretching cycle (Fig. 4.13).[73] The first four cycles of stretching to 10% beyond the muscle's resting length were found to produce some 80% of the length changes (Fig. 4.13).[73] This is a familiar experience to anyone who exercises: after the first stretch, the second and third stretches become progressively easier, until the stretching reaches plateau at which there is little further elongation.

Oscillatory stretches

Much like cyclical stretching, oscillatory stretching may help to reduce discomfort during treatment. Such a technique involves the use of fine oscillatory stretches superimposed at the end-range (see Fig. 4.12 above). These oscillations are performed at the resonant frequency of the joint.[68] An example of such a technique is to have the patient sitting on the treatment table with the lower leg hanging freely off the edge. The leg can then be oscillated like a pendulum into cycles of flexion and extension. Generally, these oscillations are of very fine amplitude and are unlike the ballistic type of stretching.

ACTIVE MUSCLE STRETCHING

Another common method of stretching the muscle–tendon unit is to utilize the patient's own force of muscle contraction.[80–82] To differentiate this from passive forms of stretching, the term 'active stretching' is employed. This type of stretching is achieved by passively stretching the muscle to its full length. The patient is then instructed to contract the muscle in its lengthened position (Fig. 4.14). The contracting muscle provides the tensile forces needed to elongate its own connective tissue elements. This phase is followed by a relaxation phase during which the muscle is passively stretched to a new length. The whole process of contraction and relaxation is repeated several times, the muscle being elongated further in each successive cycle. Normally,

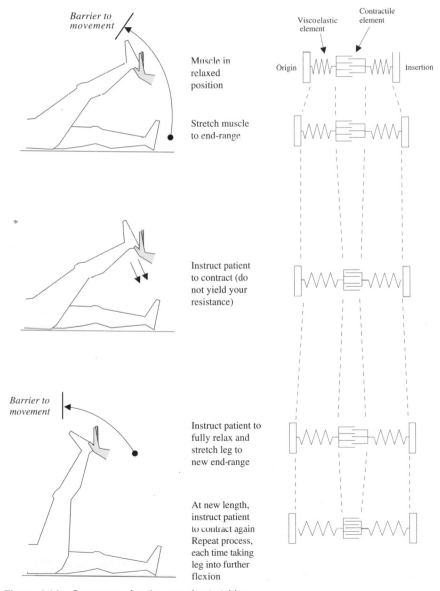

Figure 4.14   Sequence of active muscle stretching.

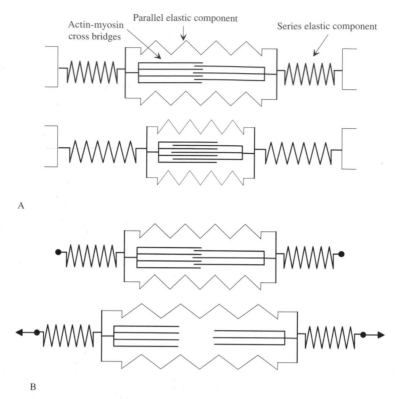

Figure 4.15 Changes in the connective tissue element of the muscle during muscle contraction and passive stretching. (A) During contraction, the series elastic components are under tension and elongate, whilst the tension in the parallel elastic components is reduced. (B) During passive stretching, both the parallel and elastic components are under tension. However, the less stiff parallel fibres will elongate more than the series component. (The separation between the actin and myosin has been exaggerated.)

three to four cycles are enough to stretch the muscle maximally. The elongation in the muscle following active stretches is solely a biomechanical event related to the viscoelastic properties of the muscle–tendon unit; these changes are not neurologically induced (see Section 2).

Passive and active muscle stretching are not comparable processes. For example, during the contraction phase in active stretching, the series elastic components are exclusively stretched. Only during the passive phase are the parallel elastic components (such as myofascia; see Fig. 4.15) also stretched. Active stretching will be ineffective at stretching non-muscular structures such as ligaments and joint capsules. For example, if the leg is raised with the knee fully

extended (hip flexion), the hamstrings will be put under tension, but the capsule and ligaments of the hip joint will not. If the capsule of the hip is to be stretched, the stretch on the hamstrings must be removed by flexing the knee (Fig. 4.16).

Many of the rules that govern passive stretching are applicable to active stretching. It has been recommended that the contraction phase should last for a period of at least 15 seconds to allow creep changes to take place. It should be noted that passive stretching should be over a similar period to allow the parallel elastic components to undergo similar changes. Although maximal muscle contraction is usually recommended, in my own experience even low-force contraction will produce length changes. In this situation, a

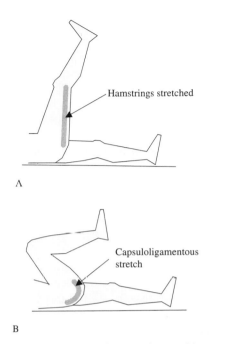

Figure 4.16   Active and passive muscle stretching are not entirely comparable. (A) Active muscle stretching. (B) Passive stretching for the hip joint.

trade-off can be achieved by reducing the force of contraction for longer periods of contraction.

Combined loading of the limb before the initiation of contraction will promote stretches of different muscle compartments. For example, if the deltoid muscle is being actively stretched, priming the muscle by external or internal rotation of the shoulder will promote a stretch in different origins and insertions of the muscle.

Active muscle stretching can be also used on spinal muscles. For example, spinal rotators can be stretched by fully rotating the patient's thorax in one direction and instructing the patient to return to the midline against resistance. The patient is then instructed to fully relax, and the trunk is further rotated. This process can be repeated several times, the spine being taken into further rotation during each cycle.

Contraindications to active stretching

In the first few days after muscle damage, active stretching should be avoided altogether. In active

stretching, there are two opposing forces working in the muscle: elongation, coupled with muscle contraction/shortening. These two opposing forces, may be the cause of some damage to the muscle, similar to those seen during isometric and eccentric contractions.[20,23,83] These stretches may closely imitate the original mode of injury, prising apart the repair site.[22]

Following a strain injury to the muscle, the initial physiological response is inflammation and oedema rather than structural shortening.[20] In the early stages after injury, passive pump techniques should be used to help disperse oedema. Once the muscle has regained its tensile strength, active or passive stretching can be added, the force of stretching or contraction being graded to the progressive increase in the muscle's tensile strength. High-force contractions and stretching should be postponed until the late regeneration and remodelling phases.

RESTORING FULL RANGE MOVEMENT: POSSIBLE MECHANISMS FOR LONG-TERM CHANGES

There are three possible mechanism by which tissue elongation can be achieved: creep deformation, plasticity and a remodelling process. The question arises of which of these mechanisms accounts for the long-term changes brought about by manual stretching. Creep deformation is an unlikely mechanism as it results in only a transient elongation. Normal turnover of connective tissue (which is a slow remodelling process) in fully healed or normal but shortened tissue is also a slow process that may take from a few month to years. This could not explain the rapid length changes that may take place after only several weeks of stretching. Plasticity is therefore a more plausible mechanism for long-term changes.

It has been proposed that stretching causes minor rupture of the collagen fibres, leaving free 'end-points'.[74] These end-points initiate an inflammatory response and the subsequent synthesis of collagen by the fibroblasts. This collagen is deposited to reunite the end-points, culmi-

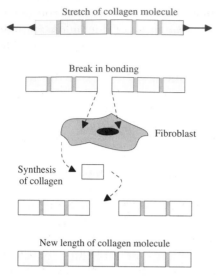

Stretch of collagen molecule

Break in bonding

Fibroblast

Synthesis of collagen

New length of collagen molecule

Figure 4.17 Stretching may cause plastic changes and lead to a remodelling process with permanent elongation of the tissue.

nating in elongation of the fibres (Fig. 4.17). This process can be likened to adding more links to a chain.

In normal but short healthy tissue, minor plasticity may be related to the elongation and failure of normal collagen fibres (such as stretching during exercise to 'improve flexibility'). In tissue that has shortened as a result of injury, permanent length changes may occur from damage to abnormal cross-links or adhesions.

In muscle tissue, length changes may also be associated with tissue damage and repair. This process may be similar to muscle damage seen following unaccustomed exercise where there is splitting of the muscle cell and damage to the muscle's connective tissue elements.[84] This is a fast adaptation process. Length changes in muscle can also take place by an increase in the number and length of the sarcomeres. The latter is gradual adaptive length change not associated with muscle damage.

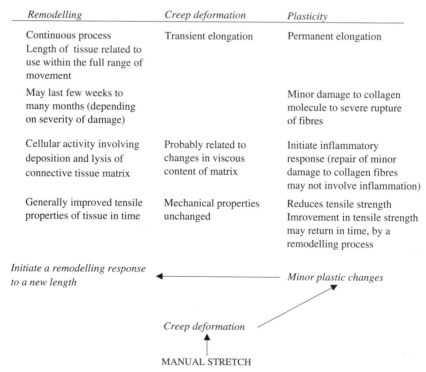

Remodelling	Creep deformation	Plasticity
Continuous process Length of tissue related to use within the full range of movement	Transient elongation	Permanent elongation
May last few weeks to many months (depending on severity of damage)		Minor damage to collagen molecule to severe rupture of fibres
Cellular activity involving deposition and lysis of connective tissue matrix	Probably related to changes in viscous content of matrix	Initiate inflammatory response (repair of minor damage to collagen fibres may not involve inflammation)
Generally improved tensile properties of tissue in time	Mechanical properties unchanged	Reduces tensile strength Imrovement in tensile strength may return in time, by a remodelling process

Initiate a remodelling response to a new length ← *Minor plastic changes*

Creep deformation

MANUAL STRETCH

Figure 4.18 Remodelling, creep deformation and plasticity: possible mechanisms for long-term length changes following stretching.

The fine damage to collagen or muscle fibres will initiate a repair response and subsequent remodelling process. The maintenance of long-term changes in length are probably related to the background mechanical environment providing the stimulus for remodelling in the lengthened position. This environment is maintained by the repetitive stretching during manipulation or by the patient's return to full range movement. For example, the improvement in cervical movement obtained by stretching will be maintained by the patient's return to daily activities, for example, turning their head when parking a car. This sequence of events and differences between remodelling, creep deformation and plasticity are depicted in Fig. 4.18.

Minor plasticity can be viewed as a positive therapeutic objective in which the tissue is encouraged to adapt by 'controlled damage'.

The adverse reaction

Stretching is associated with varying degrees of plasticity and tissue damage, and is therefore the source of the adverse reaction seen after treatment. This response can range from mild stiffness and discomfort to severe pain. The magnitude of the adverse reaction is probably proportional to the severity of damage (plasticity) that has taken place. Positively, stretching results in minor discomfort or stiffness following treatment without loss of mechanical strength of the tissue. Negatively stretching may produce a severe painful reaction and reduce the tissue's mechanical strength. Several variables – the velocity, force and frequency of stretching – will determine the severity of response. The higher the force and velocity, the greater the potential for damage. Also, if stretching is applied too frequently, it will prevent the resolution of inflammation between successive episodes of stretching, which could lead to chronic inflammation and low-level repair. How to reduce the potential for severe adverse reactions has been discussed throughout this chapter.

5

Changes in tissue fluid dynamics

The human body can be viewed as a vast network of fluid systems comprising blood, interstitial fluid, lymph, synovial fluid and cerebrospinal fluid. Normal flow within the tissues and exchange between fluid compartments is essential for homeostasis and the health of the body. Via these fluid systems various nutrients such as oxygen, glucose, fats, proteins, vitamins and minerals, are delivered to the body's tissues. The removal of tissue products from the cellular environment is also dependent on normal flow.[85,86] Any impediment to normal flow leads to stagnation, resulting in impaired tissue nutrition, viability and repair.

This chapter aims to identify the manual techniques that may facilitate fluid flow in the body. Conditions that may be helped by manual stimulation of flow are inflammation following physical trauma, oedema, joint effusion and ischaemic conditions such as nerve root irritation, or compartment syndrome in muscle. There are three main fluid systems that will be affected by manipulation:

- blood
- lymph
- synovial fluid.

An important drive for flow is the fluctuating pressure gradients within and between the different fluid compartments (fluid moving from high-pressure to low-pressure areas). These are generated by pulsatile mechanisms such as the heart pump, the muscle pump, the respiratory pump and movement. Flow can be augmented by techniques that imitate these fluid-propelling mechanisms. Manipulation can also affect fluid flow by reducing structural obstructions within the tissue. The structural influences of manipulation were discussed in the previous chapter.

GENERAL PHYSIOLOGICAL CONSIDERATIONS

In the average human adult, some 60% of the body weight is water. About one third of the total body water is extracellular, and the remaining two-thirds is intracellular. The extracellular fluid is composed of two compartments: the circulating blood plasma and the interstitial fluid, which includes the lymphatic system.[87] In essence, most of the manual work directed at this level aims to promote the movement of fluids and their contents from one compartment to the other (Fig. 5.1).

The term 'hydrokinetic transport' will be used to denote the movement of fluids along pressure gradients, aided by mechanical forces. The fluid tension within the tissue is termed 'hydrostatic pressure'. Not all fluid flow is by hydrokinetic transport: fluids also move across compartments by diffusion, which does not require mechanical force or external energy. This chapter will focus on hydrokinetic mechanisms, which are most likely to be influenced by manipulation.

FLOW THROUGH THE INTERSTITIUM

The intersititium is the anatomical space surrounding the cells. This space is composed of an intricate collagen, water and GAG matrix (see Ch. 2). The interstitium is believed to have very fine channels, forming a porous medium. Through these channels, blood-borne products pass from the capillaries to the venules and lymph system (Fig. 5.2).[21,88] The fluid passing through this matrix is composed essentially of dissolved proteins and their support fluid. Fluid filtrate from the capillary is reabsorbed by the venous or lymph system. Proteins are largely removed from the interstitium via the lymph.

Fluid flow through the intersitium is affected by osmotic and hydrostatic gradients, and protein transport is affected by hydrostatic pressure and the concentration of proteins in the

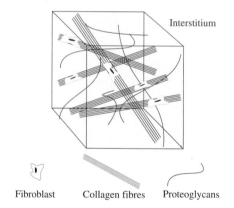

Figure 5.2 The interstitium has a porous structure with microscopic channels for the movement of fluids and solutes.

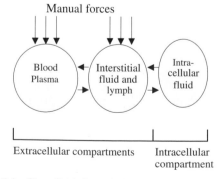

Figure 5.1 The effect of manipulation on fluid flow in the different tissue compartments.

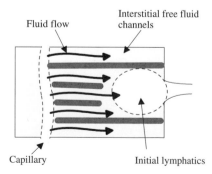

tissue.[88] Small solutes such as oxygen and sugars move through the interstitium by diffusive transport. Generally, as the solutes become larger, hydrokinetic transport becomes more important as it 'pushes' the solutes through the micropores in the matrix. This is brought about by the periodic deformation of the tissue by mechanical stresses, for example, during movement. Macromolecules such as proteins, hormones, enzymes and waste products, are almost exclusively transported by hydrokinetic transport.[21,89] This transport may also be the stimulus for increased cellular metabolism. Hydrokinetic transport is important for tissue growth and healing and may be impaired in the absence of mechanical stress in immobilized tissues.[21]

IMPEDIMENTS TO FLOW

Obstruction and impediment to flow can arise from intrinsic factors within the tissue itself or extrinsic factors that exert inward pressure (Fig. 5.3). An example of intrinsic pressure is that created by the inflammatory process within the tissue soma/parenchyma, or the commonly observed increased fluid pressure in muscle tissue after exertion (see Section 2 on muscle tone).[90] Extrinsic factors affecting fluid dynamics arise from surrounding tissues that impinge upon the tissue's vascular and lymphatic supply and drainage.

Fluid flow is markedly affected by small changes in the diameter of the vessel.[85,87] For example, a 10% decrease in the diameter of the tube will lead to a 33% reduction in flow. This demonstrates how even a small swelling around the tissue will severely reduce the flow in that area.

Intrinsic factors impeding flow

The inflammatory process is one of the most

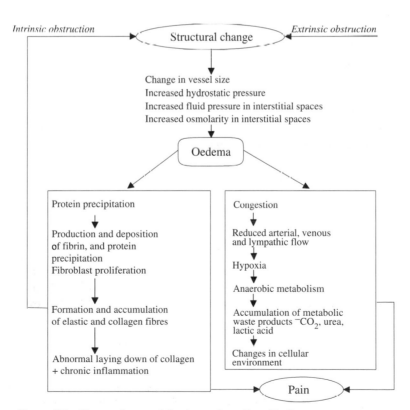

Figure 5.3   Tissue changes following an impediment to flow.

frequent causes of impeded flow in and around damaged tissue. Chemical vasodilators are released, causing dilatation of venules and capillaries. There is also a local increase in the permeability of the blood vessels, with reduced flow velocity. This leads to the formation of local oedema and stasis with reduced delivery of nutrients to the area as well as decreased drainage of metabolic byproducts. This internal distension may impede tissue healing and quality of repair, resulting in contractures, adhesions and excessive cross-link formation.[85] Fortunately, the acute inflammatory reaction does not always follow such a chronic destructive pathway, and most injuries throughout life heal spontaneously and without complications. Even in such normal events, manipulation could have a role in reducing the level of discomfort and pain as well as aiding the quality and rate of repair (see Ch. 3).

Extrinsic impediments to flow

Extrinsic impediment to flow can arise from local structural abnormalities, as well as gross musculoskeletal and fascial distortions. An example of external structural obstruction is nerve root irritation as a result of disc injury.[91,92] The causes of nerve root damage are largely related to distortion and compression of the venous plexus within the intervertebral foramen by inflammatory oedema. This leads to venous stasis and ischaemia of local tissue, and subsequently to pathological changes within and around the nerve root, including perineural and intraneural fibrosis, oedema of the nerve root and focal demyelination. Another example of such local obstruction is in carpal tunnel syndrome, where the otherwise healthy median nerve is compressed by swelling of surrounding damaged tissue. In these conditions, there is a double 'irrigation' problem: one arising from stasis of the injured tissue itself (carpal tunnel soft tissues), the other from the reduced flow to adjacent normal tissue (nerve tissue), resulting in neural ischaemia. In both examples, the symptomatic picture is related to both the primary lesioned tissue (e.g. the disc) and the secondary lesioned tissue (e.g. the nerve), which lie in close anatomical proximity. The success of treating such a multiple lesion largely relies on reducing the swelling in the primary lesion. The question that arises during diagnosis is whether the impinging lesion is of *solid material* (solid condition) such as scar tissue, adhesion or contracture which can be manually stretched, or is an *oedematous structure* (soft condition), which will respond to pump-like techniques. This concept will be discussed more fully below.

RESPONSE OF BLOOD FLOW TO MANUAL LOADING

Internal and external forces such as muscle contraction and intermittent compression will affect blood flow in the muscle.[93] There are two principal forms of manipulation that use this mechanism to facilitate flow through muscle:

- active muscle pump techniques
- passive muscle pump techniques.

ACTIVE PUMP TECHNIQUES

Active pump techniques activate the muscle's own fluid-propelling mechanism, i.e. rhythmic muscle contraction. Active pump techniques can be used in conditions where the muscle is ischaemic, oedematous or inflamed. The advantage of this type of technique over the passive pump technique is the depth of drainage produced by the muscle contraction, which will affect flow extensively throughout the muscle. In comparison, massage or effluerage may be more 'superficial' and may not reach the core of the muscle, especially in large-bellied muscles (such as the calf muscles). Over my years in practice, I have often used these techniques for treating various muscle conditions. On many occasions, where passive techniques did nothing to relieve pain, only active pump techniques produced a positive response. The response is often quite dramatic, with immediate pain relief lasting far beyond the cessation of treatment.

MUSCLE CONTRACTION AND BLOOD FLOW

Blood flow within muscle is strongly affected during muscle contractions.[94,95] Changes in the rate of flow are an immediate adaptation to the increased metabolic activity of the contracting muscle. This increase in flow is partly due to changes in the permeability and dilatation of the muscle capillaries (hyperaemia), and the mechanical compression of the venules. Hyperaemia is controlled by the sympathetic supply to the blood vessels in the muscle and by vasoactive chemicals, for example histamine, that are released locally during muscle activity.[87] These local changes in the capillary bed are transient, persisting for a short period after muscle activity (varying with the level of activity).[87,96]

Depending on fibre arrangement, there is during contraction a pressure cascade from the centre to the periphery that propels venous blood away from the muscle (Fig. 5.4).[97,98] The compression of the capillaries by contraction results in decreased flow to the muscle (Fig. 5.5), the degree of which is related to the level of intramuscular fluid pressure. The resistance to flow rises in proportion to the force of contraction.[99,100] At about 10% of maximum voluntary contraction (MVC), flow will start reducing and at 70% MVC it is totally abolished (arterial to venous).[87,101] During the relaxation phase, the intramuscular fluid pressure drops, the flow resuming and being enhanced (owing to hyperaemia).[94,102] It has

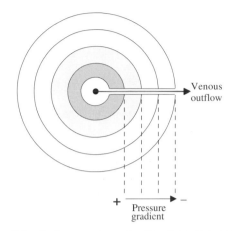

Figure 5.4   During muscle contraction, there is a pressure gradient with central high pressure (dark shading) to peripheral low pressure (light shading). Venous flow is down the pressure gradient.

been demonstrated that, in a rhythmically contracting muscle, blood flow may increase 30-fold.[87]

PRINCIPLES OF THE TECHNIQUES

Active pump techniques are derived from the principles described above. These techniques use intermittent muscle contraction to increase blood flow in muscles. Muscle pump technique can be initiated by instructing the patient to oscillate the limb freely between two spatial positions (Fig. 5.6). The therapist's hands guide the range of movement and also provide a stop to the

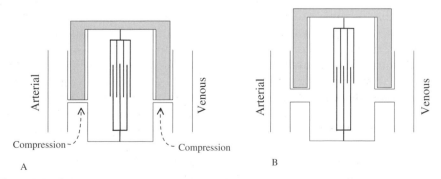

Figure 5.5   Schematic representation of blood flow during muscle contraction and relaxation. (A) During muscle contraction, blood flow is reduced as a result of increased intramuscular pressure. (B) Blood flow in the muscle resumes during muscle relaxation.

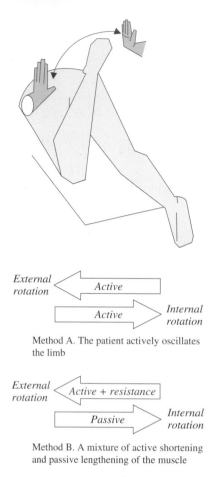

Method A. The patient actively oscillates the limb

Method B. A mixture of active shortening and passive lengthening of the muscle

Figure 5.6 Examples of different active muscle pump techniques.

patient's limb, which prevents the patient using his or her own muscles to 'brake' the movement at end-range. Alternatively, the muscle pump can be initiated by the patient performing a shortening contraction (to maximize the intramuscular pressure), followed by a full relaxation and passive elongation of the muscle to the perceived resting position of the muscle (to minimize intramuscular pressure and increase flow). For example, in the piriformis muscle, an active muscle pump can be produced by the patient actively externally rotating the leg against low-level resistance. Afterwards, the patient is instructed to relax fully, and the limb is passively rotated into internal rotation (Fig. 5.6). This procedure can be repeated several times, but

without allowing fatigue or pain to develop; feedback can be provided by the patient.

Active pump techniques can be used in conjunction with passive techniques. This pattern can be used in conditions in which intramuscular pressure is not responding to passive techniques. A few cycles of muscle contraction against resistance can be used to initiate vascular changes (hyperaemia), which will transiently 'open up' the blood flow in the muscle. Passive technique immediately follows, taking advantage of the hyperaemia and the increase in flow. This could improve the effectiveness of the passive pump techniques. The alternate use of active and passive pump techniques can be repeated several times during the treatment, i.e. a repetition of active pump, followed by a few cycles of passive pump, technique, repeating this pattern several times (Fig. 5.7).

Frequency and force

Some indication of the frequency and force of contraction of active pump techniques can be derived from studies of blood flow in the quadriceps muscle during and following rhythmic exercise. Such a study also demonstrated a similar pattern of reduced flow in the contraction phase and increased flow in the relaxation phase.[103] Each phase lasted for 2 seconds and the exercise was carried out for a period of 6 minutes. As the force of contraction increased, so did blood flow, up to 50% of the maximal contraction force. Beyond that level, the increase in flow was small. Hyperaemia lasting for about 2.5 minutes was observed immediately on cessation of the exercise.

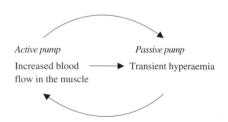

Figure 5.7 Alternate use of active and passive muscle pump techniques can be a potent stimulus to blood flow.

Generally, the force of contraction during active pump techniques should be minimal. Full forceful contraction may further fatigue the muscle and increase pain.

Pattern of contraction

Maximum intramuscular pressure is achieved when the muscle is contracting in its shortened position, but less so when the muscle is contracting in its lengthened position.[100,102] This implies that a more effective muscle pump may be achieved with the muscle activated during a shortening contraction (concentric) rather than when the muscle is contracted while being elongated (eccentric). It is also more efficient when the muscle is not fully stretched. During the relaxation phase, the muscle is positioned at its resting length (which is related to the joint neutral or resting position).[86,104] In this position, the intramuscular pressure and resistance to flow are minimal.

PASSIVE MUSCLE PUMP TECHNIQUES

External compression can also be used for enhancing flow in a relaxed muscle. The vascular events during external compression are probably similar to those during muscle contraction. There is partial collapse of blood and lymph vessels as the muscle is deformed by compression, which will encourage venous flow but partially reduce arterial flow.[105] The emptying of the venous vessels will form an arterial–venous pressure gradient. During decompression, flow resumes and may even transiently increase as a result of the arterial–venous pressure gradient.

Intermittent external compression

Rhythmic intermittent compression is often used to increase the flow in muscles.[106] The techniques involve rhythmic cycles of manual compression and decompression of the muscle. It is important that the compressive force is high enough to be transmitted deep into the muscle. Low forces will not deform the muscle and may affect only flow in superficial structures, such as skin. Ideally, the muscle should be in its resting position to allow free flow during manipulation.

Static and rhythmic stretching

Transverse or longitudinal slow stretching is often used to facilitate blood flow in muscle. However, the techniques employed may not be as effective as intermittent compression or rhythmic stretching (see below). This is due to an increase in intramuscular pressure during stretching which leads to a reduction of blood flow.[100] In contrast, rhythmic stretching may produce some flow changes in muscle, although these may not be as effective as in rhythmic intermittent compression. The force of stretching is an important element in facilitating flow. Generally, the intramuscular fluid pressure rises in proportion to the force of stretching (however, these forces should be applied in a dynamic rather than static manner).[99,100]

Other manual techniques

In a study comparing hacking and kneading techniques, it was found that vigorous hacking increased muscle blood flow,[107] the increase lasting for 10 minutes after the cessation of hacking. Kneading the muscle produced an insignificant change in blood flow. The difference between the two forms of manipulation has been attributed to the more traumatic effect of hacking, causing cellular damage followed by the release of local vasodilators. It has also been suggested that the increase in flow results from reflex muscle contraction during hacking. Although the tendon reflex can be activated by manual tapping, this is highly unlikely to be the source of the increase in flow as the contraction produced by the tendon reflex is very weak in comparison with normal muscular activity. Hence, the results obtained during hacking must be attributed to local hyperaemia. It is not clear why kneading, which included compression, squeezing and friction, did not produce any significant change in flow, as it has been demonstrated that external compression using an inflatable cuff does increase blood flow.[106]

Variables such as rate, force, frequency and direction all probably play an important part in enhancing flow. The characteristics of some of these variables may be deduced from the effect of external compression on lymph formation and drainage (see below). The possible potency of different forms of manipulation on flow through the muscle is demonstrated in Figure 5.8. However, more research is needed to establish which of these techniques is most effective.

RESPONSE OF LYMPH FLOW TO MANUAL LOADING

Intermittent tissue compression, and passive and active movement, provide a potent stimulus for lymph formation and flow.[108,109] Increased lymphatic flow indicates an increase in diffusion and filtration between the blood compartment and the interstitial/lymph compartment. Manipulation, whether active or passive, can encourage such flow. This movement may aid the passage of blood-borne nutrients to damaged tissue and the drainage of metabolic waste products. Improving lymph flow in and around a

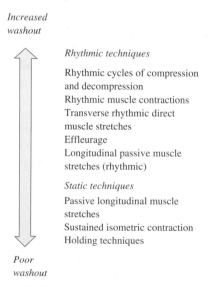

Figure 5.8 The possible potency of different manual techniques on muscle blood flow.

damaged tissue will facilitate the healing process and may help to reduce pain. The importance of increasing flow at the site of damage has been demonstrated in a study of post-traumatic fracture of the ankle. In this study, joint mobility, pain and oedema were examined following intermittent pneumatic compression (which is very similar to intermittent manual compression).[110,111] The study group consisted of patients with a distal fracture of the lower limb. After removal of the plaster cast, each patient in the study group received 75 minutes of intermittent compression for 5 consecutive days. The control group did not receive any treatment. Ankle joint mobility increased by 11.9° in the study group but by only 1.0° in the control group. This increase in the range of joint movement occurred in the absence of any kind of joint articulation. The study group also experienced significantly greater pain relief. The reduction in oedema was 170 ml in the study group but only 15 ml in the control group.

VARIABLES AFFECTING LYMPH FLOW

Several variables will affect lymph flow:

- frequency of drainage
- external force
- pattern of drainage
- passive and active movement.

Frequency of drainage

The draining and filling of lymph vessels is rate and time dependent, and is therefore influenced by the frequency of external compression.[108,109] Lymph flow increases dramatically as the frequency of intermittent compression is increased. The duration of both compression and decompression will have an effect on flow rate. During the decompression period, there is refilling of the lymphatic vessels (this filling rate can be demonstrated by stroking the veins of the forearm in from distal to proximal). However, the length of time of tissue compression does not change the rate of flow. Once lymph is squeezed out of the vessel's lumen, there is no need for further compression.

Although increasing the rate of intermittent compression will result in an increase in flow, rapid loading in damaged tissue could result in further tissue damage. This may be caused by the sudden increase in local hydrostatic pressure exceeding the damaged vessel's tensile strength. Such a mechanism of damage is analogous to stepping slowly or rapidly on a juice carton. If the carton is compressed slowly, the juice will seep out of the straw hole without the carton rupturing. However, if the carton is loaded rapidly, it will burst, as the pressure inside exceeds the rate at which the juice can flow out.

External force

Increasing the force of compression also increases the flow rate. Increasing the pressure leads to compression of greater numbers of lymphatics, which were not affected at lower compression pressures (Fig. 5.9). The stronger the compression used, the larger and deeper the area of tissue being compressed, affecting a larger number of lymphatics (as opposed to higher compression pushing more fluid from the same lymphatics).[108,109] The main lymphatic ducts possess an intrinsic propulsion system activated by smooth muscle,[112] and are not affected to the same extent as by external compression. The lymphatic ducts are affected by mechanical events, such as the thoracic pump and gravity.

Pattern of drainage

The movement of lymph is along a pressure gradient, from a high- to a low-pressure area.[99,113] During treatment, this tendency can be enhanced by creating low-pressure areas proximal to the area of damage into which lymph can be drained. The proximal lymphatics are drained before the distal ones (Fig. 5.10).[113] Clearing the lymphatics in the proximal area creates a reservoir into which the oedema from the affected area can be emptied (in some texts these reservoirs are also called 'lymphsheds'). Reducing the hydrostatic pressure in the proximal area provides less resistance to flow 'down the line', thus protecting the tissue from further damage.[99,113] Direct effleurage and compression of damaged tissue will lead to an increase in hydrostatic pressure and result in further microtrauma. Figure 5.10 demonstrates this pattern of drainage in the upper limb. In localized inflammation or oedema, a similar proximal to distal sequence can be used (sometimes these techniques are called 'deep friction'). Drainage is initiated at the periphery of the swelling to provide a local reservoir (Fig. 5.11). Subsequently, drainage is applied to the swollen area itself, slowly increasing the force of compression. Periods of destress should be also included in such a treatment.

The flow in the main ducts is usually (although not always) directed towards the heart and is affected by gravity. Thus, manual drainage should ideally be towards the heart. Lifting the limb may further facilitate the drainage.

Passive and active movement

Passive and active movement of a limb will increase its lymph flow.[108,112] Movement of the limb produces drainage by affecting both deep and superficial tissues. Movement can be likened to three-dimensional drainage. In comparison, massage tends to influence superficial lympha-

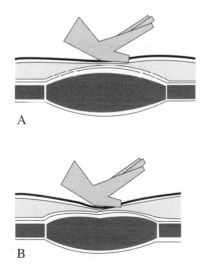

A

B

Figure 5.9 The effect of compression force on fluid dynamics. (A) Low force will deform only a superficial area of the tissue, resulting in unchanged drainage. (B) Increasing the pressure deforms deeper tissues, thus increasing lymphatic drainage.

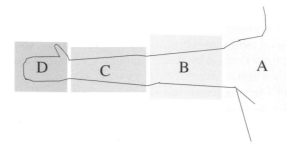

Drainage of the whole upper extremity and its division into compartments:
A, deltoid-scapula; B, upper arm; C, forearm; D, hand. Sequence of drainage–
Starting at A, then B–A, C–B–A and finally D–C–B–A.

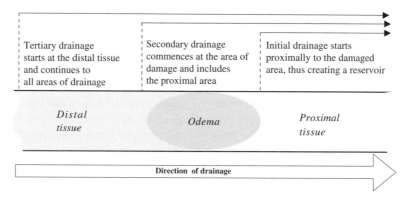

Figure 5.10   Sequence of lymphatic drainage.

tics and can be likened to two-dimensional drainage. Animal studies have demonstrated that flexion of the metatarsal–phalangeal joint produces an increase in lymph flow comparable to that from skin massage.[114] To make drainage deeper and more effective, treatment should combine movement with massage techniques. Rhythmic muscle contraction will also influence lymph flow within the contracting muscle and can be used as described above in active pump techniques.[108,112,115]

RESPONSE OF SYNOVIAL FLUID TO MANUAL LOADING

To some extent, synovial fluid physiology is largely forgotten in manual therapy, yet the mechanisms of its formation and clearance from the joint cavity are strongly affected by joint movement.[27] This response to movement suggests that manipulation could be a potent therapeutic tool in treating different joint pathologies.[27,49]

GENERAL CONSIDERATIONS

Synovial fluid has a viscous consistency, much like egg white. Its main role is to lubricate the moving articular and synovial surfaces, as well as supplying nutrients to much of the avascular articular cartilage.[27,116] Synovial fluid is a dialysate of blood plasma, containing some protein (hyaluronate) and mucin which is synthesized by cells in the synovial lining. The synovial lining is thin, between one and three cells deep, and rests on loose connective tissue, backed by muscle, fibrous capsule, tendon or fat. Some 80% of the

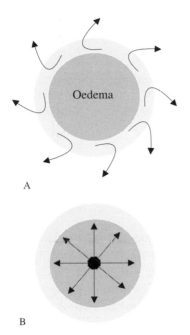

A

B

Figure 5.11 Sequence of deep draining of local inflammation and oedema. (A) Drainage is initiated at the periphery of the oedematous area to create a local reservoir. (B) Once the periphery of the oedematous area has been 'opened', deep draining of the area can proceed.

surface is cellular, and the remaining area, the interstitial space, is a highly permeable matrix. This matrix allows the flux of nutrients and fluids between the joint cavity and extra-articular

fluid systems. The synovial lining has a highly vascular component that is superficial in relation to the joint cavity. This proximity contributes to the ease of exchange of nutrients and metabolic byproducts.

Trans-synovial pump

The movement of fluids and synovial products into and out of the joint is dependent on joint motion. Movement, be it active or passive, produces intra-articular pressure fluctuations (Fig. 5.12). Flexion of the joint increases the intra-articular pressure, which drives fluid out of the joint. Extension reduces intra-articular pressure, increasing the net movement of fluids into the joint cavity.[116,117] This flow, brought about by movement, is called the trans-synovial pump effect. The speed at which fluids move in and out of the joint is called the clearance rate. Part of the trans-synovial effect relates to changes in periarticular vascular and lymphatic flow (Fig. 5.13).[116] Movement will stimulate lymphatic drainage and blood flow around the joint, the latter being important for the formation of synovial fluid. Drainage of the joint is primarily via the synovial lymph system and to a lesser extent via capillaries and venules. For example, intra-articular proteins are removed exclusively via the synovial lymphatics.

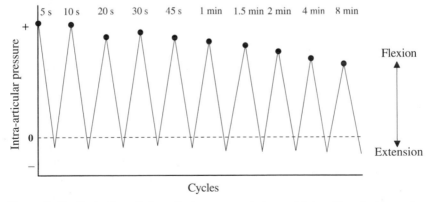

Figure 5.12 Reduction of intra-articular pressure between joint positions before and after flexion during repeated runs from 90° to 30°. Note the overall decline in pressure with the knee joint held for progressively longer periods in full flexion (30°). The time above each cycle indicates the duration of full flexion. (After Nade & Newbold 1983 with permission from the Physiological Society.[117])

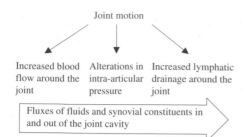

Figure 5.13 The trans-synovial pump.

Cartilage nutrition

Because articular cartilage has no direct supply route from the underlying bone, the nutrition and viability of the chondrocytes are totally dependent on synovial fluid (Fig. 5.14). The supply of nutrients to the cartilage is partly by diffusion and partly by hydrokinetic transport. This transport is aided by movement, which produces smearing and agitation of the synovial fluid on the cartilage surface.[119,20]

Nutritional transport to the articular cartilage occurs over a relatively long distance and via different tissues. Different joint pathologies that alter the structure and function of the synovial membrane and the capsule will impede this transport.[118] This could lead to damage and death of the chondrocytes and the subsequent degeneration of the hyaline matrix.

MOTION, JOINT DAMAGE AND HEALING

Continuous passive motion has been shown to promote the healing of minor cartilage damage in experimental animals (Fig. 5.15). It has been shown that small defects in the articular surfaces of mobilized joints can heal by hyaline rather than fibrocartilage, as is found in immobilized animals. Continuous passive mobilization was substantially more effective at promoting such changes, being better even than active intermittent mobilization, in which the animal was allowed to move freely.[51] New formation of cartilage has been shown to take place in intra-articular periosteal grafts under continuous passive motion conditions. Even slight degrees of motion or intermittent pressure are sufficient to stimulate the production of small amounts of cartilage.[48]

Clinically, passive motion is used in the treatment of various musculoskeletal conditions. Passive motion into full extension has been shown significantly to improve the range of movement and to reduce pain in spinal disc injuries.[121] A treatment of 20–30 minutes produces immediate positive changes (the frequency used being 10 cycles/min). Continuous passive

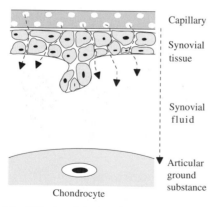

Figure 5.14 Diffusion distance of nutrients from synovial capillary to chondrocyte. (After Fassbender 1987.[118])

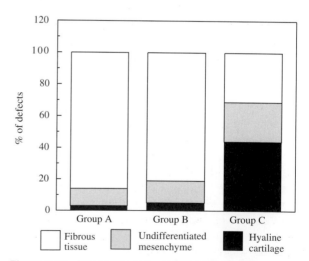

Figure 5.15 The nature of the repairing tissue after articular cartilage damage in adult animals. Group A was immobilized, group B was given intermittent active motion and group C was treated with continuous passive motion (36 animals in each group). (After Salter et al 1980[51]).

movement is also used postoperatively to facilitate joint healing.[122] This form of treatment tends to reduce the recovery time and pain level and improve the quality of repair.

Passive motion and clearance rate

Increased synovial fluid volume and pressure will give rise to sensations of tension, pain and limitation of movement. This may be accompanied by muscular weakness brought on by reflex inhibition, which is initiated by joint afferents (see Section 2). Above a critical effusion pressure, there may be (but is not always) an impairment of synovial blood flow, reducing the movement of nutrients in and waste products out of the joint cavity. For example, increased intra-articular pressure in osteoarthritic knees has been shown to reduce synovial blood flow; this may contribute to joint anoxia and cartilage damage in chronic arthritis.[123] In animal models, increased intracapsular pressure reduces femoral head blood flow.[124] Similarly, ischaemia of the femoral epiphysis in children suffering from septic arthritis of the hip was shown to be reduced by joint aspiration.[125]

Passive motion of joints may help to reduce effusion and facilitate the rate of healing.[126] Passive cycles of flexion and extension of the spine have been shown to produce pressure fluctuations within the facet joints.[127] When saline was injected into the facet joint artificially to increase intra-articular pressure, cycles of active and passive motion caused a drop in this pressure. This effect was greater when the manipulation was specific to the effused joint. Passive motion has been shown to facilitate the transport of synovial fluid contents (in and out of the joint). In one such study, a tracer substance was used to study the nutrition of the anterior cruciate ligament under conditions of continuous passive motion and rest. It was found that, in knees that were passively moved, the clearance rate of the tracer was so rapid that it did not have sufficient time to diffuse into the ligament.[128] Other studies have shown the benefits of passive motion in reducing haemarthrosis.[129] After 1 week of treatment with passive motion, there

was a significant decrease in the amount of blood in the treated, compared with the untreated joints. Passive motion was shown also to affect the outcome of septic arthritis, leading to less damage of the articular cartilage.[130] This was attributed to the effective removal of the damaging lysosomal enzymes by accelerated clearance rate.

Manual techniques influencing the trans-synovial flow

The healing of joints may be aided by gentle passive motion within the *pain-free* range of movement. In these conditions manipulation is in the form of *movement rather than stretching* (Fig. 5.16). An example of passive movement is passive pendular swings of the lower legs while the patient is sitting on the edge of the table. In this position, the knee can be freely swung into cycles of flexion and extension. Five minutes of swinging produces some 600–800 cycles, which is almost equivalent to the number of knee flexion/extension cycles in 0.5 km of walking. Similar pendular movements can be produced in the glenohumeral joint by swinging the free

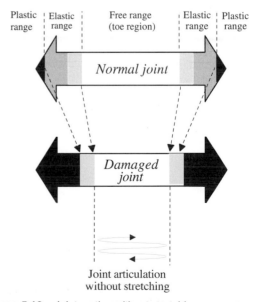

Figure 5.16 Joint motion without stretching.

hanging arm into cycles of flexion and extension. Spinal joints can be oscillated when the patient is lying prone and the pelvis is rocked in rotation around the long axis of the body.

Most joints in the body can be articulated using oscillatory movements. These oscillations can be maintained with little effort for up to 15–20 minutes. I have frequently used passive oscillation without the need for needle aspiration and without adverse reactions. The response to treatment is usually immediate, the patient being able to weight-bear or use the limb with less discomfort. This form of manipulation is usually introduced immediately after injury. For a full description of oscillatory type technique see Lederman (1991).[68]

Effluerage and elevation of the limb can be added to further promote drainage of the limb. These techniques can be used to create low-pressure reservoirs and stimulate local flow around the capsule.

The use of rest, ice, compression and elevation (RICE) is recommended to aid the healing of sprained joints. Perhaps the acronym RICE should be changed to MICE, to include the beneficial use of motion immediately after the injury. It should again be emphasized that excessive motion and mechanical stress can traumatize the tissue and may be detrimental to its long-term viability (Fig. 5.17).[47]

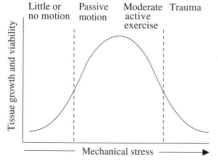

Figure 5.17 Qualitative effects of low, moderate and high mechanical stress on tissue growth and viability. (After Hargens & Akeson 1986 with permission from Springer-Verlag.[21])

TREATMENT STRATEGIES AT THE LOCAL TISSUE ORGANIZATION: SOFT AND SOLID CONDITIONS

Broadly speaking, most musculoskeletal conditions can be classified as being either solid or soft conditions, or as having both qualities:

1. Soft conditions are lesions that have a water-like consistency, as in oedema and inflammation.
2. Solid conditions usually relate to longer-term changes in the tissue that are 'hard' in nature, for example, scar tissue, adhesions, contractures and shortened tissue.

Classifying tissue state into these two categories can simplify and clarify the process of matching the most effective manipulation to the patient's condition. Treatment of soft and solid conditions requires different manual techniques. A soft condition will be affected by the rhythmic compressive mode of loading, but only minimally by tensile forces. Solid conditions such as muscle shortening will benefit from stretching rather than compression or effleurage.[130] The manual consideration in treatment of the two types of lesions are further exemplified in Table 5.1.

It is possible for both conditions to be superimposed, for example in chronic joint strain with stiffness and inflammation. The stiffness in this case can be categorized as a solid condition owing to excessive cross-link formation or adhesions. The inflammation in this case is a soft condition. In a combined condition, treatment should start with managing the soft lesion as it is usually the source of pain and discomfort. Once inflammation and pain have reduced and the tissue has regained its tensile strength, stronger manipulation can commence to increase the joint's range of movement.

PAIN RELIEF BY MANIPULATION: LOCAL TISSUE MECHANISMS

One possible mechanism for the immediate pain

Table 5.1   Manual considerations in the treatment of soft and solid conditions

Physiological process	Aim of treatment	Mode of manipulation
Soft condition Inflammation Oedema Swelling Impediment to flow	To improve tissue healing and nutrition To improve fluid dynamics within the tissues	Gentle passive techniques Intermittent compression Articulation within the pain free range of movement Low stress with minimal stretching (preferably compression rather than stretching)
Deposition of collagen and remodelling process	To improve the tissue's mechanical properties To reduce adhesion and excessive cross-links formation	Initial low loading and stretching of tissue Progressive increase in loading commensurate with increase in tissue strength
Solid condition Loss of extensibility/ flexibility of tissue	To improve tissue flexibility and mechanical behaviour under loading	Medium to high-force loading Longitudinal or cross-fibre techniques Slow repetitive or sustained stretches Combined modes of loading
Adhesion and abnormal cross-link formation	To lessen adhesions and abnormal cross-links	High-force loading Longitudinal or cross-fibre techniques High-velocity loading (very dangerous, consider carefully) Slow repetitive stretches or sustained stretches.

relief seen after manipulation is related to the direct effect that manipulation has on local pain mechanisms. (Neurological and psychological pain processes are discussed in Sections 2 and 3 respectively. Section 4 gives an overview of the three organizations of pain.)

Inflammation is the most common cause of musculoskeletal pain. Non-inflammatory pain such as muscle ischaemia is discussed in Chapter 8. In inflammation, pain arises by local physiological changes that irritate the various pain-conveying fibres. There are three mechanisms to account for this irritation (Fig. 5.18):[132,133]

- *Mechanical irritation*: Inflammatory oedema causes local swelling, which increases the pressure in the tissue and irritates pain receptors.
- *Chemical irritation*: Local substances are

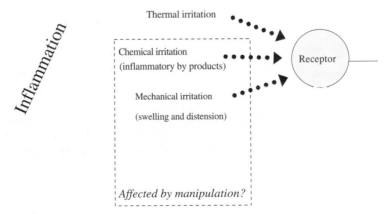

Figure 5.18   Possible role of manipulation in reducing local causes of pain. Affecting fluid flow may help to reduce chemical (inflammatory byproducts) and mechanical (swelling) irritation.

released by various cells at the site of damage, lowering the pain threshold and exciting pain receptors.

• *Thermal irritation*: The temperature at the site of damage tends to rise and excite pain receptors. Thermal irritation can be ameliorated by non-manual methods such as applying cold packs, but these treatment modalities are outside the scope of this book.

A decrease in mechanical and chemical irritation may be the source of the immediate and postmanipulation reduction of pain. Both forms of irritation will be affected by changes in local fluid dynamics. The mechanism that may underlie pain relief may be related to the potential of manipulation to increase flow in the tissue. Such changes in fluid dynamics would affect the level of inflammatory byproducts at the site of damage, thus reducing the chemical source of irritation. Manipulation may also help to disperse the inflammatory oedema (swelling), helping therefore to reduce the mechanical irritation at the site of injury. It would be expected that following manipulation, chemical and mechanical irritation would gradually return by build-up of inflammatory by-products and mechanical pressure.

Techniques that can influence flow at the site of damage have been discussed extensively in Chapter 5. These techniques are intermittent compression, massage, effleurage and passive movement. Inflammation and oedema in muscle may be reduced by passive and low-level active techniques. Stretching, high-velocity thrusts (adjustments) and holding techniques (functional, sacrocranial) will have little or no effect on local fluid dynamics and are therefore unlikely to affect pain mechanisms at the tissue level of organization. This goes back to the principle of soft and solid condition discussed in Table 5.1 above.

6

Overview and summary of Section 1

This section has discussed the relationship between different manual events and a tissue's physiological response. Changing the many variables of manipulation, such as mode, rate, force, duration and repetition, will promote different physiological responses in the designated tissue.

Three areas in which manipulation can be used at the level of tissue organization have been identified: facilitating repair processes, influencing the structure and mechanical behaviour of tissues, and affecting fluid dynamics.

In the early stages of the repair process, passive techniques can be used providing they are of low force and amplitude, are within the pain-free range of movement and do not disturb the integrity of the repair. Manual techniques that may facilitate the repair process are rhythmic or oscillatory techniques. Repetition of the manual event is very important for a successful outcome: single, static and transient manual events will have little effect on the repair process. Strong forces, and high-amplitude or high-velocity manual events are contraindicated during the early stages of the repair process, as these techniques will disrupt the repair site, resulting in further damage and a reduced quality of repair. Stretching can be introduced later in the repair process when the tissue has gained some mechanical strength. However, the force and amplitude of stretching must not exceed the tissue's mechanical strength or physiological range.

Structural and mechanical changes in the state of the tissue can be achieved with passive stretches. Depending on the level of mobility and extendibility of the tissue, the amplitude and force of stretching need to be adjusted accordingly. Since elongation of a tissue is time and rate dependent, slow, static stretches are recommended to effectively lengthen a shortened tissue. Repetition of stretching is also important for mechanical remodelling and plastic changes to take place. Active stretching can be useful in elongating shortened muscle. However, non-muscular structures such as ligaments or joints capsules will not be affected by active stretching. Single, short-duration and explosive-type stretching will have little effect on tissue elongation.

Fluid dynamics are best influenced by rhythmic cyclical events that mimic the body's own pump mechanisms. These techniques are very important in conditions where there is inflammation and where stretching is contra-indicated. Techniques that may help to propel fluids are intermittent compression, effleurage and rhythmic active and passive movement. Rhythmic joint movement will also affect the formation and clearance rate of synovial fluid. Here, too, repetition is important for a successful outcome. Single, static and short-lasting manual events will have little effect on fluid dynamics.

Manipulation may also affect pain processes by its influence on fluid flow. Such flow changes may help reduce swelling and the build-up of inflammatory byproducts.

References

1. Zachazewski J E 1989 Improving flexibility. In: Rosemary M, Scully R M, Barnes R (eds) Physical therapy. JB Lippincott, London
2. Carlstedt C A, Nordin M 1989 Biomechanics of tendons and ligaments. In: Nordin M, Frankel V H (eds) Basic biomechanics of the musculoskeletal system. Lea & Febiger, London, ch. 3, p 698–738
3. Aukland K, Nicolaysen G 1981 Interstitial fluid volume: local regulatory mechanisms. Physiological Reviews 61: 3
4. Hukins D W L, Kirby M C, Sikoryn T A, Aspden R M, Cox A J 1990 Comparison of structure, mechanical properties, and function of lumbar spinal ligaments. Spine 15: 8
5. Nakagawa H, Mikawa Y, Watanabe R 1994 Elastin in the posterior longitudinal ligament and spinal dura. Spine 19(19): 2164–2169
6. Gray's Anatomy 1980 Williams P L, Warwick K (eds) Churchill Livingstone, London
7. Bornstein P 1980 The biosynthesis, secretion and processing of procollagen. In: Viidik A, Vuust J (eds) Biology of collagen. Academic Press, London, p 61–75
8. Viidik A, Danielsen C C, Oxlund H 1982 On fundamental and phenomenological models, structure and mechanical properties of collagen, elastin and glycosaminoglycan complex. Biorheology 19: 437–451
9. Woodhead-Galloway J 1981 The body as engineer. New Scientist 18: 772–775
10. Millington P F, Wilkinson R 1983 Skin. Cambridge University Press, Cambridge
11. Arem A J, Madden J W 1976 Effects of stress on healing wounds. I. Intermittent noncyclical tension. Journal of Surgical Research 20: 93–102
12. Cooper J H 1969 Histochemical observation on the elastic sheath: elastofibril system of the dermis. Journal of Investigative Dermatology 52: 169–176
13. Hunter G 1994 Specific soft tissue mobilisation in the treatment of soft tissue lesions. Physiotherapy 80(1): 15–21
14. Madden J W, DeVore G, Arem A J 1977 A rational postoperative management program for metacarpophalangeal joint implant arthroplasty. Journal of Hand Surgery 2: 358–366

15. Madden J W, Peacock E E 1971 Studies on the biology of collagen during wound healing. III. Dynamic metabolism of scar collagen and remodelling of dermal wounds. Annals of Surgery 174: 511–520

16. Tillman L J, Cummings G S 1993 Biology mechanisms of connective tissue mutability. In: Currier D P, Nelson R M (eds) Dynamics of human biological tissue. F A Davies. Philadelphia,Ch. 1, p 1–44

17. Baur P S, Parks D H 1983 The myofibroblast anchoring strand: the fibronectin connection in wound healing and possible loci of collagen fibril assembly. Journal of Trauma 23: 853–862

18. Madden J W, Peacock E E 1968 Studies on the biology of collagen during wound healing. I. Rate of collagen synthesis and deposition in cutaneous wounds of the rat. Surgery 64(1): 288–294

19. Hunt T K, Van Winkle W 1979 Normal repair. In: Hunt T K, Dunphy J E (eds) Fundamentals of wound management. Appleton-Century-Crofts, New York, ch. 1, p 2–67

20. Byrnes W C, Clarkson P M 1986 Delayed onset muscle soreness and training. Clinics in Sports Medicine 5(3): 605–614

21. Hargens A R, Akeson W H 1986 Stress effects on tissue nutrition and viability. In: Hargens A R (ed.) Tissue nutrition and viability. Springer-Verlag, New York

22. Lennox C M E 1993 Muscle injuries. In: McLatchie G R, Lennox C M E (eds) Soft tissues: trauma and sports injuries. Butterworth Heinemann, London, p 83–103

23. Newham D J, Jones D A, Tolfree S E J, Edwards R H T 1986 Skeletal muscle damage: a study of isotope uptake, enzyme efflux and pain after stepping. European Journal of Applied Physiology 55: 106–112

24. Allbrook D B, Baker W deC, Kirkaldy-Willis W H 1966 Muscle regeneration in experimental animals and in man. Journal of Bone and Joint Surgery 48B(1): 153–169

25. Allbrook D 1981 Skeletal muscle regeneration. Muscle and Nerve 4: 234–245

26. Newham D J 1991 Skeletal muscle pain and excercise. Physiotherapy 77(1): 66–70

27. Akeson W H, Amiel D, Woo S L-Y 1987 Physiology and therapeutic value of passive motion. In: Joint loading: Helminen H J, Kivaranka I, Tammi M (eds) Biology and health of articular structures. John Wright , Bristol, 375–394

28. Akeson W H, Amiel D, Woo S L 1980 Immobility effects on synovial joints: the pathomechanics of joint contracture. Biorheology 17: 95–110

29. Akeson W H, Amiel D, Mechanic G L, Woo S L-Y, Harwood F L, Hamer M L 1977 Collagen cross-linking alterations in joint contractures: changes in the reducible cross-links in periarticular connective tissue collagen after nine weeks of immobilization. Connective Tissue Research 5: 15–19

30. Frank C, Akeson W H, Woo S L-Y, Amiel D, Coutts R D 1984 Physiology and therapeutic value of passive joint motion. Clinical Orthopaedics and Related Research 185: 113–125

31. Amiel D, Woo S L-Y, Harwood F, Akeson W H 1982 The effect of immobilization on collagen turnover in connective tissue: a biochemical-biomechanical correlation. Acta Orthopaedica Scandinavica 53: 325–332

32. Harwood F L, Amiel D 1990 Differential metabolic responses of periarticular ligaments and tendons to joint immobilization. American Physiological Society, p 1687–1691

33. Vailas A C, Tipton C M, Matthes R D, Gart M 1981 Physical activity and its influence on the repair process of medial collateral ligament. Connective Tissue Research 9: 25–31

34. Gelberman R H, Manske P R, Akeson W H, Woo S L-Y, Lundborg G, Amiel D 1986 Flexor tendon repair. Journal of Orthopaedic Research 4: 119–128

35. Gossman M R, Sahrmann S A, Rose S J 1982 Review of length associated changes in muscle. Physical Therapy 62(12): 1799–1808

36. Evans E B, Eggers G W N, Butler J K, Blumel J 1960 Experimental immobilisation and remobilisation of rat knee joints. Journal of Bone and Joint Surgery 42(A)(5): 737–758

37. Enneking W F, Horowitz M 1972 The intra-articular effect of immobilization on the human knee. Journal of Bone and Joint Surgery 54(A)(5): 973–985

38. Finsterbush A, Frankl U, Mann G 1989 Fat pad adhesion to partially torn anterior cruciate ligament: a cause of knee locking. American Journal of Sports Medicine 17(1): 92–95

39. Cummings G S, Tillman L J 1993 Remodelling of dense connective tissue in normal adult tissues. In: Currier D P, Nelson R M (eds) Dynamics of human biological tissue. F A Davies, Philadelphia, ch. 2, p 45–73

40. Forrester J C, Zederfeldt B H, Hayes T L, Hunt T K 1970 Wolff's law in relation to the healing of skin wounds. Journal of Trauma 10(9): 770–780

41. Peacock E E, Van Winkle W 1976 Wound repair, 2nd edn. W B Saunders, Philadelphia

42. Rudolph R 1980 Contraction and control of contraction. World Journal of Surgery 4: 279–287

43. Hunt T K 1979 Disorders of repair and their management. In: Hunt T K, Dunphy J E (eds). Fundamentals of wound management. Appleton-Century-Crofts, New York, Ch. 2, p 68–168

44. Rizk T E, Christopher R P, Pinals R S, Higgins C, Frix R 1983 Adhesive capsulitis (frozen shoulder): a new approach to its management. Archives of Physical Medicine and Medical Rehabilitation 64: 29–33

45. Farkas L G, McCain W G, Sweeny P et al 1973 An experimental study of the changes following silastic rod preparation of new tendon sheath and subsequent tendon grafting. British Journal of Surgery 55: 1149–1158

46. Hunt T K, Banda M J, Silver I A 1985 Cell interactions in post-traumatic fibrosis. Clinical Symposium 114: 128–149

47. Gelberman R H, Menon J, Gonsalves M, Akeson W H 1980 The effects of mobilization on vascularisation of healing flexor tendons in dogs. Clinical Orthopaedics 153: 283–289

48. Viidik A 1970 Functional properties of collagenous tissue. Review of Connective Tissue Research 6: 144–149

49. Lowther D A 1985 The effect of compression and tension on the behaviour of connective tissue. In: Glasgow E F, Twomey L T, Scull E R, Kleynhans A M, Idczek R M (eds) Aspects of manipulative therapy. Churchill Livingstone, London, p 16–22

50. Magonne T, DeWitt M T, Handeley C J et al 1984 In vitro responses of chondrocytes to mechanical loading: the effect of short term mechanical tension. Connective Tissue Research 12: 98–109

51. Salter R B, Simmonds D F, Malcolm B W, Rumble E J, MacMichael D, Clements N D 1980 The biological effect of continuous passive motion on the healing of full-thickness defects in articular cartilage. Journal of Bone and Joint Surgery 62(A)(8): 1232–1251

52. Convery F R, Akeson W H, Keown G H 1972 The repair of large osteochondral defects: an experimental study in horses. Clinical Orthopaedics and Related Research 82: 253–262

53. Fronek J, Frank C, Amiel D, Woo S L-Y, Coutts R D, Akeson W H 1983 The effect of intermittent passive motion (IMP) in the healing of medial collateral ligament. Proceedings of the Orthopaedic Research Society 8: 31 (abstract)

54. Leivseth G, Torstensson J, Reikeras O 1989 The effect of passive muscle stretching in osteoarthritis of the hip. Clinical Science 76: 113–117

55. Sadoshima J-I, Seigo I 1993 Mechanical stretch rapidly activates multiple signal tranduction pathways in cardiac myocytes: potential involvement of an autocrine/paracrine mechanism. EMBO Journal 12(4): 1681–1692

56. Leung D Y M, Glagov S, Mathews M B 1977 A new in vitro system for studying cell response to mechanical stimulation. Experimental Cellular Research 109: 285–298

57. Palmar R M, Reeds P J, Lobley G E, Smith R H 1981 The effect of intermittent changes in tension on protein and collagen synthesis in isolated rabbit muscle. Biomechanics Journal 198. 491–498

58. Strickland J W, Glogovac V 1980 Digital function following flexor tendon repair in zone 2: a comparison of immobilization and controlled passive motion techniques. Journal of Hand Surgery 5(6): 537–543

59. Gelberman R H, Woo S L-Y, Lothringer K, Akeson W H, Amiel D 1982 Effects of early intermittent passive mobilization on healing canine flexor tendons. Journal of Hand Surgery 7(2): 170–175

60. Savio S L-Y, Gelberman R H, Cobb N G, Amiel D, Lotheringer K, Akeson W H 1981 The importance of controlled passive mobilization on flexor tendon healing. Acta Orthopaedica Scandinavica 52: 615–622

61. Gelberman R H, Amiel D, Gonsalves M, Woo S, Akeson W H 1981 The influence of protected passive mobilization on the healing of flexor tendons: a biochemical and microangiographic study. Hand 13(2): 120–128

62. Takai S et al 1991 The effect of frequency and duration of controlled passive mobilization on tendon healing. Journal of Orthopaedic Research 9(5): 705–713

63. Lagrana N A et al 1983 Effect of mechanical load in wound healing. Annals of Plastic Surgery 10: 200–208

64. Arnold J, Madden J W 1976 Effects of stress on healing wounds. I. Intermittent noncyclical tension. Journal of Surgical Research 29: 93–102

65. Light N D, Baily A J 1980 Molecular structure and stabilization of the collagen fibre. In: Viidik A, Vuust J (eds) Biology of collagen. Academic Press, London, p 15–38

66. Dunn M G, Silver F H 1983 Viscoelastic behaviour of human connective tissues: relative contribution of viscous and elastic components. Connective Tissue Research 12: 59–70

67. LaBan M M 1962 Collagen tissue: implication of its response to stress in vitro. Archives of Physical Medicine and Rehabilitation 43: 461–466

68. Lederman E 1997 Harmonic technique. Churchill Livingstone, Edinburgh (in press)

69. Warren C G, Lehman J F, Koblanski 1976 Heat and stretch procedure: an evaluation using rat tail tendon. Archives of Physical Medical and Rehabilitation 57: 122–126

70. Viidik A 1987 Properties of tendon and ligaments. In: Handbook of Bioengineering. McGraw-Hill, New York

71. Viidik A 1980 Interdependence between structure and function in collagenous tissues. In: Viidik A, Vuust J (eds) Biology of collagen. Academic Press, London, p 257–280

72. Jamison C E, Marangoni R D, Glaser A A 1968 Viscoelastic properties of soft tissue by discrete model characterization. Journal of Biomechanics 1: 33–46

73. Taylor D C, Dalton J D, Seaber A V, Garrett W E 1990 Viscoelastic properties of muscle-tendon units: the biomechanical effects of stretching. American Journal of Sports Medicine 18(3): 300–309

74. Rigby B J 1964 The effect of mechanical extension upon the thermal stability of collagen. Biochimica et Biophysica Acta 79: 634–636

75. Rigby B J, Hirai N, Spikes J D 1959 The mechanical behavior of rat tail tendon. Journal of General Physiology 43: 265–283

76. Light K E, Nuzik S, Personius W 1984 Low load prolonged stretch vs. high load brief stretch in treating knee contractures. Physical Therapy 64: 330–333

77. Gainsbury J M 1985 High velocity thrust and pathophysiology of segmental dysfunction. In: Glasgow E F, Twomey L T, Scull E R, Kleynhans A M, Idczek A M (eds) Aspects of manipulative therapy. Churchill Livingstone, London, p 87–93

78. Holmes M H, Lai W M, Mow V C 1986 Compression effects on cartilage permeability. In: Hargens A R (ed.) Tissue nutrition and viability. Springer-Verlag, New York

79. Bandy W D, Irion J M 1994 The effect of time on static stretch on the flexibility of the hamstring muscles. Physical Therapy 74(9): 845–850

80. Hartley-O'Brian S J 1980 Six mobilization exercises for active range of hip flexion. Research Quarterly 5(4): 625–635

81. Sady S P, Wortman M, Blanke D 1982 Flexibility training: ballistic, static or proprioceptive neuromuscular facilitation. Archives of Physical Medicine and Rehabilitation 63: 261–263

82. Tanigawa M C 1972 Comparison of the hold relax procedure and passive mobilization on increasing muscle length. Physical Therapy 52(7): 725–735

83. Bobbet M F, Hollander P A, Huijing P A 1986 Factors in delayed onset muscular soreness of man. Medicine and Science in Sports and Exercise 18(1): 75–81

84. Ebbeling C B, Clarkson P M 1989 Exercise–induced muscle damage and adaptation. Sports Medicine 7: 207–234

85. Zink J G 1977 Respiratory and circulatory care: the conceptual model. Osteopathic Annals 5(3): 108–112

86. Barclay J K 1995 Introduction to the functional unit. Symposium: Mechanisms which control VO_2 near VO_2max. Medicine and Science in Sports and Exercise 27(1): 35–36

87. Ganong W F 1981 Dynamics of blood and lymph flow. In: Review of medical physiology. Lang Medical Publication, California, ch. 30, p 470–484

88. Meyer F A 1986 Distribution and transport of fluids as related to tissue structure. In: Hargens A R (ed.) Tissue nutrition and viability. Springer-Verlag, New York

89. Maroudas A 1986 Mechanisms of fluid transport in cartilaginous tissues. In: Hargens A R (ed.) Tissue nutrition and viability. Springer-Verlag, New York

90. Konno S, Kikiuchi S, Nagaosa Y 1994 The relationship between intramuscular pressure of paraspinal muscles and lower back pain. Spine 19(19): 2186–2189

91. Hoyland J A, Freemont A J, Jayson M I V 1989 Intervertebral foramen venous obstruction: a cause of periradicular obstruction? Spine 14(6): 558–568

92. Toyone T, Takahashi K, Kitahara H, Yamagata M, Murakami M, Moriya H 1993 Visualisation of symptomatic nerve root: prospective study of contrast enhanced MRI in patients with lumbar disc herniation. Journal of Bone and Joint Surgery 75(B)(4): 529–533

93. Gardner A M N, Fox R H, Lawrence C, Bunker T D, Ling R S M, MacEachern A G 1990 Reduction of post-traumatic swelling and compartment pressure by impulse compression of the foot. Journal of Bone and Joint Surgery 72(B): 810–815

94. Brechue W F, Ameredes B T, Barclay J K, Stainsby W N 1995 Blood flow and pressure relationship which determine VO_2max. Medicine and Science in Sports and Exercise 27(1): 37–42

95. Dodd S L, Powers S K, Crawford M P 1994 Tension development and duty cycle affect Qpeak and VO_2peak in contracting muscle. Medicine and Science in Sports and Exercise 26(8): 997–1002

96. Kamm R D 1987 Flow through collapsible tubes. In: Handbook of Bioengineering. McGraw-Hill, New York

97. Kirkebo A, Wisnes A 1982 Regional tissue fluid pressure in rat calf muscle during sustained contraction or stretch. Acta Physiologica Scandinavica 114: 551–556

98. Hill A V 1948 The pressure developed in muscle during contraction. Journal of Physiology 107: 518–526

99. Gillham L 1994 Lymphoedema and physiotherapists: control not cure. Physiotherapy 80(12): 835–843

100. Sejersted O M et al 1984 Intramuscular fluid pressure during isometric contraction of human skeletal muscle. Journal of Applied Physiology 56(2): 287–295

101. Petrofsky J S, Hendershot D M 1984 The interrelationship between blood pressure, intramuscular pressure, and isometric endurance in fast and slow twitch muscle in the cat. European Journal of Applied Physiology 53: 106–111

102. Sejersted O M, Hargens A R 1986 Regional pressure and nutrition of skeletal muscle during isometric contraction. In: Hargens A R (ed.) Tissue nutrition and viability. Springer-Verlag, New York

103. Walloe L, Wesche J 1988 Time course and magnitude of blood flow changes in the human quadriceps muscles during and following rhythmic exercise. Journal of Physiology 405: 257–273

104. Weiner G, Styf J, Nakhostine M, Gershuni D H 1994 Effects of ankle position and a plaster cast on intramuscular pressure in the human leg. Journal of Bone and Joint Surgery 76(A)(10): 1476–1481

105. Laughlin M H 1987 Skeletal muscle blood flow capacity: role of muscle pump in exercise hyperemia. American Journal of Physiology 253(22): 993–1004

106. Airaksinen O, Kolari P J 1990 Post-exercise blood lactate removal and surface electromyography as models of the effects of intermittent pneumatic compression treatment on muscle tissue. Manual Medicine 5: 162–165

107. Hovind H, Nielsen S L 1974 Effect of massage on blood flow in skeletal muscle. Scandinavian Journal of Rehabilitation Medicine 6: 74–77

108. McGeown J G, McHale N G, Thornbury K D 1987 The role of external compression and movement in lymph propulsion in the sheep hind limb. Journal of Physiology 387: 83–93

109. McGeown J G, McHale N G, Thornbury K D 1988 Effects of varying patterns of external compression on lymph flow in the hind limb of the anaesthetized sheep. Journal of Physiology 397: 449–457

110. Airaksinen O 1989 Changes in post–traumatic ankle joint mobility, pain and oedema following intermittent pneumatic compression therapy. Archives of Physical Medicine and Rehabilitation 70(4): 341–344

111. Airaksinen O, Partanen K, Kolari P J, Soimakallio S 1991 Intermittent pneumatic compression therapy in posttraumatic lower limb edema: computed tomography and clinical measurements. Archives of Physical Medicine and Rehabilitation 72(9): 667–670

112. Schmid-Schonbein G W 1990 Microlymphatics and lymph flow. Physiological Review 70(4): 987–1028

113. Mason M 1993 The treatment of lymphoedema by complex physical therapy. Australian Journal of Physiotherapy 39: 41–45

114. Calnan J S, Pflug J J, Reis N D, Taylor L M 1970 Lymphatic pressures and the flow of lymph. British Journal of Plastic Surgery 23: 305–317

115. Skalak T C, Schmid-Schonbein G W, Zweifach B W 1986 Lymph transport in skeletal muscle. In: Hargens A R (ed.) Tissue nutrition and viability. Springer-Verlag, New York

116. Levick J R 1987 Synovial fluid and trans–synovial flow in stationary and moving normal joints. In: Helminen H J, Kivaranki I, Tammi M (eds) Joint loading: biology and health of articular structures. John Wright, Bristol, p 149–186

117. Nade S, Newbold P J 1983 Factors determining the level and changes in intra-articular pressure in the knee joint of the dog. Journal of Physiology 338: 21–36

118. Fassbender H G 1987 Significance of endogenous and exogenous mechanisms in the development of osteoarthritis. In: Helminen H J et al (eds) Joint loading: biology and health of articular structures. John Wright, Bristol

119. Maroudas A 1970 Distribution and diffusion of solutes in articular cartilage. Biophysical Journal 10

120. Maroudas A, Bullough P, Swanson S A V 1968 The permeability of articular cartilage. Journal of Bone and Joint Surgery 50(B)(1): 166–177

121. McKenzie R A 1994 Mechanical diagnosis and therapy

for disorders of the low back. In: Twomey L T, Taylor J R (eds) Physical therapy of the low back. Churchill Livingstone, London, p 171–196

122. Korcok M 1981 Motion, not immobility, advocated for healing synovial joints. Journal of the American Medical Association 246(18): 2005–2006

123. Geborek P, Moritz U, Wollheim F A 1989 Joint capsular stiffness in knee arthritis. Relationship to intraarticular volume, hydrostatic pressures, and extensor muscle function. Journal of Rheumatology 16(10): 1351–1358

124. Vegter J, Klopper PJ 1991 Effects of intracapsular hyperpressure on femoral head blood flow. Laser Doppler flowmetry in dogs. Acta Orthopaedica Scandinavica 64(4): 337–341

125. Hasegawa Y, Ito H 1991 Intracapsular pressure in hip synovitis in children. Acta Orthopaedica Scandinavica 62(4): 333–336

126. Twomey L T, Taylor J R 1994 Lumbar posture, movement, and mechanics. In: Twomey L T, Taylor J R (eds) Physical therapy of the lower back. Churchill Livingstone, London, p 57–92

127. Giovanelli B, Thompson E, Elvey R 1985 Measurments of variations in lumbar zygapophyseal joint intracapsular pressure: a pilot study. Australian Journal of Physiotherapy 31: 115

128. Skyhar M J, Danzig L A, Hargens A R, Akeson W H 1985 Nutrition of the anterior cruciate ligament: effects of continuous passive motion. American Journal of Sports Medicine 13(6): 415–418

129. O'Driscoll S W, Kumar A, Salter R B 1983 The effect of continuous passive motion on the clearance of haemarthrosis. Clinical Orthopaedics and Related Research 176: 305–311

130. Salter R B, Bell R S, Keeley F W 1981 The protective effect of continuous passive motion on living articular cartilage in acute septic arthritis: an experimental investigation in the rabbit. Clinical Orthopaedics 159: 223–247

131. Wiktorsson-Moller M, Oberg B, Ekstrand J, Gillquist J 1983 Effects of warming up, massage, and stretching on range of motion and muscle strength in the lower extremity. American Journal of Sports Medicine 11(4): 249–252

132. Levine J, Taiwo Y 1994 Inflammatory pain. In: Wall P D, Melzack R (eds) Textbook of pain, 3rd edn. Churchill Livingstone, London, p 45–56

133. Meyer R A, Campbell J A, Raja S 1994 Peripheral neural mechanisms of nociception. In: Wall P D, Melzack R (eds) Textbook of pain, 3rd edn. Churchill Livingstone, London, p 13–44

Neurological organization in manual therapy

7

Introduction to Section 2

This section examines the effect of manipulation on the neurological organization. In particular, it discusses the possible influences that manipulation may have on the organization of the motor system. The neurological mechanisms of pain and how they may be affected by manipulation are also examined. The autonomic nervous system will be discussed in Section 3.

The motor system's responsiveness to movement and guidance makes manual therapy one of the dominant treatment modalities for the rehabilitation and normalization of the neuromuscular system. Treatment of neuromuscular dysfunction by manual therapy can be seen in many and varied conditions. It may be in the form of normalizing abnormal muscle (motor) tone in patients with central nervous system damage, such as in stroke conditions; in treatment of the neuromuscular system in musculoskeletal injury, such as following joint or muscle injury; or in postural rehabilitation or re-education.

A FUNCTIONAL APPROACH

Throughout this section, the functional aspect of the motor system will be explored, with minimal consideration of the structural/anatomical aspect. It is the functional mechanisms of the motor system which form the basis of neurorehabilitation, as treatment ultimately relates to functional loss; detailed anatomical knowledge of the site and size of lesion rarely changes the course of treatment. Where there is damage to the central nervous system, treatment cannot mechanically correct this neural damage, but it can provide the stimulus needed for adaptation and plasticity of the healing areas.

In peripheral nerve or musculoskeletal injuries, there is direct tissue damage that is accessible to manipulation. Treatment of such injuries is largely a biomechanical event requiring a mechanical approach.[1] Its aim is to remove the mechanical pressure on the nerve or facilitate local tissue repair (see Section 1). In this case, good anatomical knowledge is essential for successful treatment. Often this type of injury is accompanied by neuromuscular abnormalities such as muscle weakness and wasting. Direct mechanical treatment of the muscle will not be sufficient to reverse these alterations: the neuromuscular connection has to be functionally stimulated for a change to take place. The role of manual therapy in facilitating this process is discussed throughout this section.

Neurological function can be viewed as the *normal relationship between stimulation, motivation, drives and needs, and the motor response* (for an explanation of these terms, see Fig. 7.1). Abnormality and dysfunction of the nervous system can be viewed as the failure of the system to respond in an appropriate way to stimulation, motivation, drives and needs (Fig. 7.2). In neurorehabilitation, the aim is to 'approximate' these differences.

In this book, the nervous system is divided into two separate organizations: the neurological (Section 2) and psychophysiological (Section 3) organizations. This is an artificial division used merely for the purpose of simplification: these organizations do not exist as distinct structural or functional entities. Motor processes are brought about by the complex interaction of the two organizations, and the nervous system should be viewed as a whole, a functional and anatomical continuum.

NEUROLOGICAL CLASSIFICATION OF MANUAL TECHNIQUES

All techniques in this section are classified in relation to their functional effect on the nervous

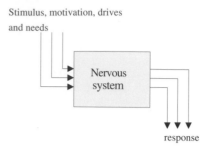

Functional model

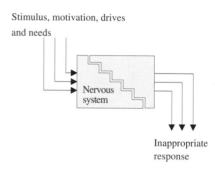

Dysfunctional model

Figure 7.1 Schematic model of function and dysfunction in the CNS. Stimulation: reflex responses, such as postural adjustments. Motivation: external and internal conditions that lead to organized behaviour. It is a force, e.g. hunger or sex, impelling the organism to act. These forces appear intermittently, vary in strength and initiate the direction and variability of behaviour.[2] Drives: internal changes induced by deprivation that promote a behaviour in the organism opposing these changes in order to reach equilibrium or homeostasis.[2] Needs: basic conditions, e.g. hunger, thirst, sex and pain avoidance, that must be satisfied for the survival of the organism or species.[2]

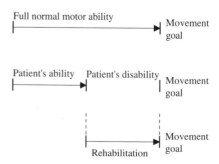

Figure 7.2 A schematic representation of the role of rehabilitation in motor disabilities. The aim of treatment is to approximate the patient's current abilities to what the therapist and patient see as a movement goal.

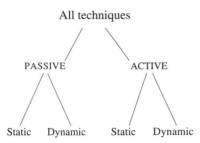

Figure 7.3 Neurological classification of manual techniques.

- dynamic techniques: involving joint movement
- static techniques: the joints are immobile.

Thus, any manual technique can be classified as being 'passive–static/dynamic' or 'active–static/dynamic'. For example, soft-tissue massage can be classified as 'passive–static'. Active techniques can be classified as 'active–static' or 'active–dynamic' depending on whether joint movement is or is not included. In Table 7.1, some common manual techniques are classified in the above manner. Throughout this section, this classification of a technique is termed 'the mode of technique', for example, passive mode, passive dynamic mode, etc. Technique factors such as rate, rhythm and force are termed 'the pattern of technique'. The relationship between the different groups of techniques and neurophysiological responses are discussed throughout this Section.

system. They are divided into two main groups (Fig. 7.3):

- active techniques: these involve voluntary movement by the patient
- passive techniques: the patient is relaxed and physically inactive.

Each of these groups is further subdivided into:

Table 7.1 Neurological classification of some common manual techniques

Passive techniques		Active techniques	
Static	Dynamic	Static	Dynamic
Soft-tissue techniques	Articulation	Active resisted techniques	Resisted joint oscillation
Effleurage	Longitudinal muscle stretching	Muscle energy techniques	Proprioceptive neuromuscular facilitation
Transverse muscle	Functional techniques		
Stretching	High-velocity manipulation		
Hacking			
Holding techniques			
Deep friction	Traction		
Inhibition	Rhythmic techniques		
Drainage techniques	Oscillatory techniques		
Cranial			
Shiatsu, acupressure and Do-in			
Strain–counterstrain			

8

The motor system

FUNCTIONAL ORGANIZATION OF THE MOTOR SYSTEM

The motor system is defined as that part of the nervous system which is involved in any physical event requiring skeletal muscle activation, such as movement, posture and the musculoskeletal aspect of behaviour and expression.

In order to understand how manipulation may affect motor processes as well as its limitations at this level, this chapter examines the functional organization of the motor system.

The motor component of the nervous system is not a discrete anatomical entity but rather an organization spanning several centres. One way of looking at the motor system is to consider its functional organization.3 Motor activity can be divided into three functional stages (Fig. 8.1):

● the executive stage: the decision-making stage
● the effector stage: the stage responsible for the enactment of movement
● sensory feedback: providing sensory information to the motor system.

These stages are not anatomically specific; for example, the executive stage is not confined to one area of the brain, but processing at this stage probably occurs at various levels within the motor system.

THE EXECUTIVE STAGE

The executive is the decision-making stage in

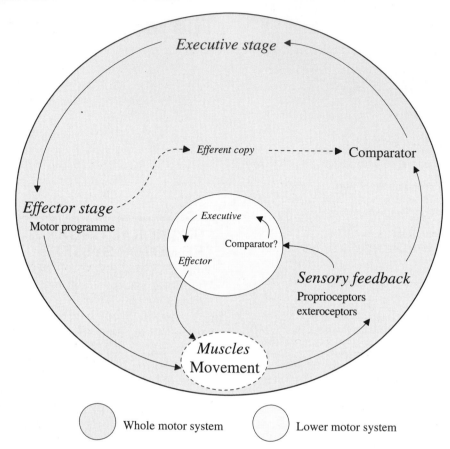

Figure 8.1 The functional organization of the motor system. The large circle represents the total or whole motor system. The small circle represents the lower parts of the motor system. Both parts of the motor system are in functional continuation. Sensory feedback to the higher executive levels is via long loops, whilst feedback to the lower motor system is via short loops.

motor processes, in which a motor event is initiated in response to volitional or reflex motor demands. At this stage, incoming sensory information is processed in relation to the eventual motor response.[4] The processing of sensory information occurs as a sequence.

It starts as *stimulus identification*, in which sensory information is analysed in relationship to ongoing motor activity. For example, lifting a glass of water from a table is preceded by the analysis of information regarding the identification of the object, its shape and size (by input arriving from vision), and the relative position of the body parts (input from proprioceptors).

Once this information is analysed, the *response selection stage* follows, during which decisions on how to respond to the sensory information are made. In the case of reaching for the cup, this will relate to which parts of the body will participate in the reaching movement (left or right arm, etc.).

Once a response has been selected, different centres are organized to carry out the movement. This stage is called *response programming stage*. It involves selecting a motor programme that will control the required movement. This includes programmes for postural adjustments to accommodate changes in the centre of gravity and the sequences of recruitment of different muscle groups.

It should be noted that processing of information at the executive stage is not always cognitive and conscious but can occur at a subconscious level.

THE EFFECTOR STAGE

The effector stage is where the execution of the motor act takes place. This is initiated by the activation of the motor programme that organizes the different centres and muscles for the desired movement. Once the chosen motor programme has been selected, a motor command is transmitted to the spinal motor centres to initiate movement. Simultaneously, information about the chosen programme is conveyed to the comparator centre (see below).

The motor programme

The motor programme is where movement and postural patterns are stored. It is probably made up of sequences of muscle activation stored in combination with sensory information from previous experiences of similar movement.[5] It is not entirely clear what form the memory has and whether it is an accurate detailed memory of the motor event or a more general, less detailed schema of movement.[6,7] The motor programme directs the motor centres on the sequence and force of muscle contractions as well as initiating postural adjustments in advance of the pursuing movement. In the case of lifting the cup off the table, such postural adjustment will precede the reaching movement in anticipation of shifts in the body's centre of gravity.[8]

A programme of movement is not centre specific but seems to be stored within different levels of the motor system. Some parts of the motor programme are situated anatomically at a very low level within the CNS: the spinal cord. In animal studies, it has been shown that a spinal animal (an animal that has only its spinal cord and not its higher centres intact) is able to produce walking patterns when placed on a treadmill.[9] I can recall my mother's story about

life on a farm: when a chicken is decapitated, it will run about for a while without its head. This implies that spinal centres are capable of storing patterns of motor activity. It is now well established that these patterns are produced by neuronal pools within the spinal cord called central pattern generators or spinal pacemakers.[9] It is believed that muscle recruitment during rhythmic activities such as running and walking is governed by spinal pattern generators. We will see later that these spinal centres are able to learn and store specific programmes even when surgically disconnected from higher centres.

THE COMPARATOR CENTRE

During motor activity, the efferent motor patterns are accompanied by a corresponding efferent copy, which is conveyed to the comparator centre (also called the correlation centre).[10] The role of this centre is to identify irregularities in movement and convey this information to the executive level.[5,11,12] The efferent copy contains a sensorimotor copy of previously stored movement patterns. Irregularities are identified by matching the efferent copy with the ongoing sensory input (Fig. 8.2).[3,13] For example, if an obstruction to movement has occurred, the increased activity from the spindles and the tendon organs would be higher then that expected from previous experience.[5] If a discrepancy is identified, it is conveyed to the executive level, where irregularities in the movement are smoothed out by moment-to-moment adjustment of the motor drive.[14]

SENSORY FEEDBACK

As the body is moving in space, the motor system needs information about internal mechanical events as well as information from the environment.[4,14] This is provided by two feedback mechanisms: *proprioceptors* provide information about internal mechanical events, whilst *exteroceptors* (vision and hearing) provide information about the environment.

Proprioceptors are found in the skin, muscles,

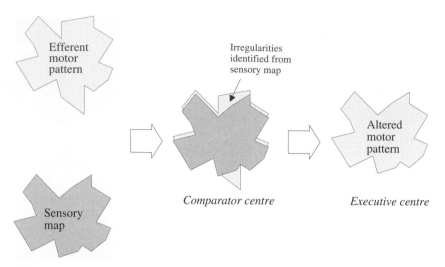

Figure 8.2   Schematic representation of the correlation centre.

tendons, ligaments and joints. When we lift an object with our hand, skin receptors signal the contact of the fingers with the object and provide information about its mass, size and texture. Further information arrives from receptors in the muscles and joints, indicating the position of the arm in space and the relationship of different body masses to each other, the speed of movement and the force of contraction. This information is integrated with visual and auditory information to provide the executive level with a sensory map of the movement.[4,14,15]

Groups of receptors neither singularly nor reflexively control the local motor output, but instead act as an ensemble providing the central motor system with a sensory map or 'picture' of movement (Fig. 8.3).[16–19] This map is dynamic, continuously moulding its shape in response to changes in position, movement and muscular activity. Proprioceptive information from one area of the body is incorporated into other streams of information from other areas. Receptors not only influence motor activity locally, but also act within the total schema of the movement.

It should be emphasized here that proprioceptors act *only in feedback* and not to control motor activity.[20] This fine distinction between feedback and control is extremely important for rehabilita-

tion of the motor system; it will be explored in more detail throughout this chapter.

The processing of proprioceptive information occurs at two principal levels within the motor system (Fig. 8.3):

1. *Conscious level*: Peripheral feedback interacts with information held in the higher centres to give conscious awareness of the position of the body in space. All groups of proprioceptors are believed to have cortical representation.[15,21,22] This can be shown by closing one's eyes and slowly flexing an index finger. With introspection, one will be aware of the joint moving, the flexor muscles contracting and the skin stretching over the joint.

2. *Automatic (reflex) level*: Not all sensory feedback reaches conscious level: many of our daily activities are performed automatically. This automatic and reflexive activity is supported by sensory information processed at a subconscious level.

CONTRIBUTION OF FEEDBACK TO MOTOR ACTIVITY

The sensory map influences the motor system in two ways (Fig. 8.3):

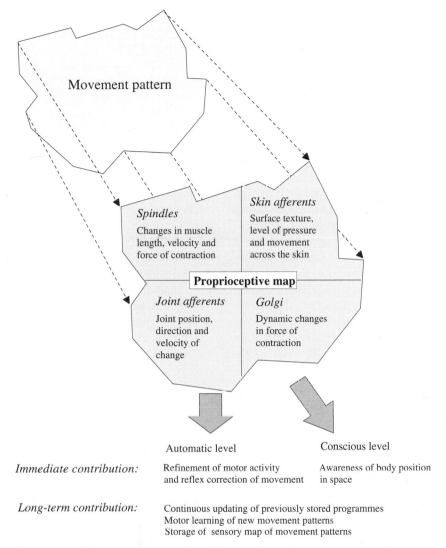

Figure 8.3 Schematic representation of the proprioceptive sensory map and its contribution to the motor system.

- adaptation/motor learning (long-term influences)
- immediate adjustments to movement (short-term influences).

SENSORY MAPS: CONTRIBUTION TO ADAPTATION/MOTOR LEARNING

Our mind is 'shaped' by our experiences and our experiences are formed by our senses. In order to learn novel movement, there must be feedback from the body. Proprioception, therefore, is important for motor learning,[12] which may be stalled if there is sensory damage. Indeed, Bobath has pointed out that the rehabilitation of stroke patients with sensory loss may be more difficult than of those with an intact system.[23]

The importance of proprioception to motor learning can be also seen in clinical conditions in which a subject loses only afferent feedback. In these circumstances, the individual is still capable of initiating motor acts that have been learned prior to injury. However, it may be difficult to modify an activity or learn a new one. In one such documented study, the subject was able to drive the car he used before his illness, but when he received a new car, he was unable to adjust to the new mechanical situation.[24]

The refinement of the prestored programmes is also dependent on proprioception, without which the motor programmes deteriorate in time and movement becomes more crude.[25] This can be demonstrated in everyday circumstances when a person attempts to carry out a physical activity that he or she has not rehearsed for a long time (e.g. cycling). A few 'goes' are usually needed to refine the stored programme. The reverse of this process can be seen in pathological conditions such as tabes dorsalis, in which damage to the dorsal horn of the spinal cord results in proprioceptive loss in the limb. Patients with this condition can still walk and move around, but, because they have lost proprioception in the limbs, they tend to have an unrefined gait. Without feedback, this pattern of walking progressively deteriorates with time. The mechanical stress produced by this gait eventually leads to degenerative joint disease (a Charcot's joint).

SENSORY MAPS: CONTRIBUTION TO IMMEDIATE ADJUSTMENTS OF MOVEMENT

On a moment-to-moment basis, proprioception is used by the ongoing motor programme to correct disturbances to movement. This process occurs at the comparator level, where feedback is continuously matched against the ongoing movement programme.

The interaction of proprioception and motor processes occurs at different levels within the motor system. By stimulating proprioceptors, the course and time of the response can be studied. The electromyogram (EMG) from the limb will show different peaks occurring at different time intervals after stimulation. The delay in the response to stimulation is called latency (in a broad sense this is a reaction time, Fig. 8.4). For a given afferent group, the further into the motor system a signal has to travel, the longer the latency of the response. To study these latencies, receptors can be artificially stimulated by different mechanical events. For example, the spindle afferents can be stimulated by a tendon tap, vibration, ramp stretch or electrical pulse. The reflex muscular response is seen on the EMG trace as being composed of up to three distinct peaks occurring at different latencies.

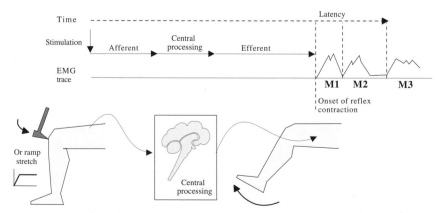

Figure 8.4 'Classical' reflex response to a single brisk stimulation of the mechanoreceptors. Note that either the M1, M2 or M3 component can be missing from the response depending on the type of stimulation used, the position of the limb and the background motor activity.

These peaks are called the M1, M2 and M3 responses (Fig. 8.4).

M1 response

The first peak (the M1 response, monosynaptic stretch reflex or tendon reflex) usually has a latency of 30–50 ms. This latency represents a short segmental pathway involving only two groups of neurons: afferent (sensory) and efferent (motor). There is some controversy over the exact function of the monosynaptic pathway. It has been suggested that, during active movement, the M1 response contributes to fast compensation for minor disturbances such as ground irregularities during walking.[26] Others have suggested that this feedback mechanism contributes to fine adjustments of muscle stiffness during walking.[8,27]

It should be noted that the short-latency reflex response is not confined to the muscle that has been stimulated: it may spread to synergistic as well as antagonistic muscle groups.[28] For example, when the biceps tendon is tapped, the reflex response spreads to muscles as far away as the pectoralis major, triceps, deltoid and hypothenar muscles.[29] Clinically, it means that, when the stretch reflex is tested in one muscle, the reflex response is diffuse throughout the limb even though the apparent reflex contraction is in only one group of muscles.

M2 response

A longer loop also feeds into a higher level within the motor system, with a latency of approximately 50–80 ms. In the lower limbs, the activity of this loop is primarily to provide information about the position of the body's centre of mass during stance and locomotion, and to contribute to postural adjustments associated with accidental slipping or hitting obstacles during walking. In the upper limbs, the feedback connections are probably related to withdrawal reflexes (such as pulling one's arm away from a hot surface).

M3 response

An even longer response with a latency exceeding 75 ms can sometimes be observed on the EMG trace.[28] This latency is often called a 'triggered reaction' and contains an element of voluntary response (one at a conscious level).[30] This response is believed to be the conscious readjustment of the limb position following the sudden reflex response. The short- and long-latency responses are not exclusive to the spindle afferents, other mechanoreceptors having influences at different levels within the motor system.[31] It should be noted that the early responses (M1 and M2) are transient (phasic), lasting only a fraction of a second.

Different forms of stimulation, the prevailing position of the limb and ongoing background motor activity will all determine the magnitude of response and which loops are activated. When the muscle is fully relaxed, sudden stretches do not always elicit the reflex response, which tends to rise with increases in the force of contraction but be abolished at high force levels.[32]

The exact role of the reflex mechanism in movement control is not fully understood. It may be that the different loops represent the course of proprioceptive feedback to different levels within the motor system. This is related to the meaning that the feedback has to the animal. If there is a small disturbance locally at a joint, it may need only local adjustments to overcome it, requiring merely short loops. If the disturbance is large, throwing the body off balance, the sensory information has to be transmitted to higher centres to provide whole-body compensation (Fig. 8.5).[33]

Strength of peripheral stimulation

The important question for manual therapists relates to how strong these reflex mechanisms are in controlling the motor system. A potent influence would indicate a strong possibility that the motor system could be influenced from the periphery. Unfortunately, these reflex influences are very mild in comparison to the responses produced by the descending motor commands.

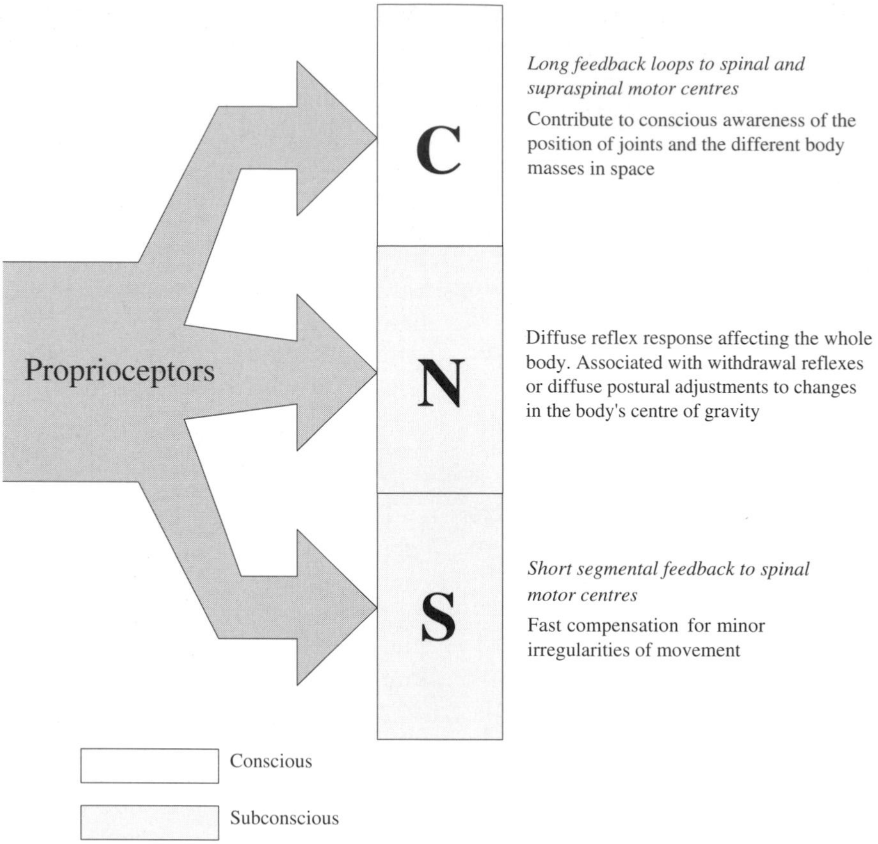

Long feedback loops to spinal and supraspinal motor centres

Contribute to conscious awareness of the position of joints and the different body masses in space

Diffuse reflex response affecting the whole body. Associated with withdrawal reflexes or diffuse postural adjustments to changes in the body's centre of gravity

Short segmental feedback to spinal motor centres

Fast compensation for minor irregularities of movement

Conscious

Subconscious

Figure 8.5 Moment-to-moment contribution of proprioceptors to the motor system.

It has been estimated that the contraction force generated by stimulation of the stretch reflex is on average 3% of the background force of contraction.[34] In animal studies, it was estimated that, of the resistance to a sudden disturbance of head movement, 10–30% was from the reflex response, but about 60% was due to the mechanical properties of the muscle.[35] This group of researchers have stated that the reflex compensation is 'modest' and results largely from the mechanical properties of the muscle, rather than from neural reflexes. Control and correction of sudden disturbances in real-life situations probably arise by the engagement of longer feedback loops that go beyond spinal centres.

EXTEROCEPTION

Vision and hearing feedback from the environment play an important role in the motor processes. Vision has a dominant role over proprioception during the early stages of motor learning. Infants who are repeatedly shown their hands while they are handling objects develop arm movement much more quickly. Similarly, young cats that are deprived of the sight of their paws will fail to develop normal walking.[36] Once a movement is memorized, however, the dominance of vision is reduced in favour of proprioception. For example, if walking or writing is a newly learned activity, it generally takes longer without vision, but once learned, one can still walk or write with the eyes shut by relying on proprioception.

The dominance of vision over proprioception has been shown in numerous studies in which subjects are instructed to handle different objects while their vision is distorted by special lenses.[36,37] Although subjects can palpate the true shape of the object, they will tend to favour the distorted image seen through the lenses. Vision also contributes to balance. When a subject's environment is manipulated without his or her knowledge, the subject tends to compensate posturally to the visual changes.[38]

Vestibular apparatus

The vestibular system is a sense organ situated within the inner ear. Functionally, it is involved in righting reflexes and balance.[13,39]

MOTOR ACTIVITY IN DELAYED AND ABSENT FEEDBACK

Delayed feedback during normal motor activity

Many motor activities do not rely on instantaneous feedback but adjust to previous sensory input. This commonly happens during rapid movements where the processing of sensory feedback is too slow to allow correction of the ongoing movement.[3,40] Delayed feedback is seen during walking, jumping, running, fast ballistic movements[41] and also fast-finger movements such as typing or playing a musical instrument. In all of these types of motor activity the preprogrammed pattern precedes the sensory feedback.[42] For example, during running and jumping, the activation of leg extensors precede, foot contact with the ground by about 150–180 ms. The correction of movement occurs only close to, or at, the termination of movement.

In the absence of feedback

Without proprioception, the motor programme can still execute skilled movements such as walking, breathing and handling objects, as was demonstrated in a subject who had total loss of leg proprioception:[43] he was able to detect error in movement although there was no feedback from the moving limb. In a different study, a subject who lost proprioception in his arm was shown to be able to produce preprogrammed (before-injury) movements of the hand and fingers with remarkable accuracy.[24] He was able to move his thumb accurately through different speed, distance and force requirements. He was, however, unable to produce fine hand movement, such as grasping a pen and writing. Without visual feedback, he was not able to maintain a constant level of muscle contraction for more than 2 seconds nor to execute long sequences of motor acts. In much the same way, monkeys who have had their sensory nerve bundle cut at its entry to the spinal cord are capable of normal climbing, balancing, playing, grooming and feeding, only was fine finger control being affected.[44,45] In a study to evaluate the role of proprioception in head movements, it was demonstrated that a monkey can rotate its head to a predetermined angle in the absence of proprioception (after cutting all the afferent fibres in the neck).[35] This ability was maintained after damage to the afferent fibres because the monkey had been trained in that particular movement prior to afferent damage. The pattern was therefore stored as a motor programme. This fact is extremely important and is often overlooked: *an intact motor system can function almost normally in the absence of proprioceptive feedback.*

Normal subjects can also produce motor activity under conditions of reduced proprioception and exteroception (vision and audition).[46] When tested for their ability to reproduce fast-finger tapping, subjects could be trained to reproduce 90% of that produced under normal conditions. One subject who had total elimination of both exteroceptive and proprioceptive feedback was able to reach 70% of the number of taps. This subject had such a total reduction of feedback that, after the tapping session, he asked whether he had tapped at all. The way in which he executed the movement was by instructing himself to 'lift and push' the finger.

The ability of the motor system to carry out movement in the absence of proprioception has been attributed to the internal feedback mechanism provided by the efferent copy and the comparator centre, providing that the movement has been prelearned before the loss of proprioception. However, in the absence of proprioception, the motor system is incapable of controlling fine or new learned movements, or of improving these movements.[9,47]

PROPRIOCEPTIVE PRIORITY AND MANIPULATION

Proprioceptors do not control the motor centres but provide information with which the motor system 'decides' on an appropriate response. If the incoming information is of low importance, the system will not modify its ongoing activity. In daily activities, a large volume of low-priority proprioceptive information is discarded as irrelevant and has no effect on motor activity.[48] For example, the fact that clothes rub against the skin while walking is low-priority information that will have no effect on ongoing motor activity.

Proprioceptive priority can change when the environment is clashing with the movement goal. Colliding with an obstacle or being pushed is high-priority proprioceptive information that will redirect the ongoing motor activity. However, the 'decision', processing and organization of the movement are by central rather than peripheral mechanisms: the system can 'choose' different movement responses, or even not to respond at all. For example, a stuntman can overcome normal postural reflexes in order to fall down a full flight of stairs.

Other examples of sensory priority can be seen in the presence of noxious stimuli. Pain is high-priority information indicating a hazard or the presence of damage. However, even in situations of extreme pain, central decision-making processes can still override nociceptive information, for example prompting the subject to run away from danger despite having an injured leg. Another example is in joint sprain and effusion. Here, joint receptors will initiate a *central*

inhibitory process directed at protecting the mechanically weakened joint from further loading. This can be also viewed as a high-priority information, but information that can also be overridden by central motor activity (see below).

The ability of the motor system to execute movement without proprioception, and assessing priorities, has far-reaching implications for the possible effect that manipulation may have on motor processes. Manipulation is a sensory event, and there is the question of whether it gives rise to high- or low-priority information and of how to change its priority. In the passive mode, most sensory information is probably of low priority with respect to any motor processes. This is primarily because, when the subject is relaxed, there are no ongoing motor events. As far as the motor system is concerned, there is nothing to 'correct' or adjust to. However, the touch experience could be and often is high-priority sensory information with profound psychological influences. These are to be considered not as motor events but as psychological responses to the manual event (see Section 3, on the psychodynamics of manipulation and the importance of proprioception in different psychological processes). To increase the manual priority in motor processes, active-type techniques are probably more effective than passive ones. This principle will be explored in Chapter 9.

RECRUITMENT OF PROPRIOCEPTORS DURING MANIPULATION

Understanding the peripheral–central relationship is important in neuromuscular rehabilitation. It provides a perspective of the potency and limitations that manual techniques will have for motor processes. This chapter looks at how the different receptors respond to the mechanical changes in the body brought about by manipulation, and whether these have any effect on motor processes.

One of the manipulator's proposed gateways to the nervous system is via activation of the body's mechanoreceptors (proprioceptors). The activity of these receptors will change in response to manual events. Many disciplines of manual therapy believe that mechanoreceptors can profoundly influence the motor system and neuromuscular activity. For example, it is believed that massage or high-velocity thrust techniques will reduce high muscle tone of neurological origin. An important question arises here of whether the motor system can be controlled from the periphery. Is it possible to reduce neuromuscular activity from the periphery by high-velocity or massage techniques? If so, which modes of manipulation will achieve this change? What are the most effective ways of influencing the motor system?

The anatomy, physiology and behaviour of proprioceptors during manipulation will now be considered. To the manual therapist, detailed receptor anatomy is not as important as their overall functional behaviour and contribution to motor processes. Manipulation does not aim to change their structure, but it aims to *modulate the information they convey to the motor system.*

GENERAL FUNCTIONAL CONSIDERATIONS

Peripheral to central communication

Mechanical events are converted by receptors into electrical signals, which are conveyed via afferent nerve fibres to the spinal cord and higher centres. The information from the periphery is transmitted centrally in the form of frequency code produced by a change in the receptor's firing rate frequency modulation.[49] Frequency modulation should not be confused with amplitude modulation (Fig. 8.6). Frequency modulation is the change in firing rate, whereas amplitude modulation varies the magnitude of each spike. *Frequency modulation implies that, even when there is no firing, the signal is still interpreted by the central nervous system as a form of information.* For example, during passive shortening of a muscle, the spindle will fall silent, i.e. there will be no firing; this 'no information' from the receptor still plays a part in the overall shape of the sensory map and the subsequent motor response.

Threshold

Each receptor has its own threshold to mechanical stimuli. Low-threshold units are activated by weak mechanical stresses, whilst high-threshold units are activated by large-magnitude events (Fig. 8.6). Any stimulus below the threshold level will not stimulate the target neuron. The sensitivity of the receptor is not fixed, and its threshold level can change. For example, inflam-

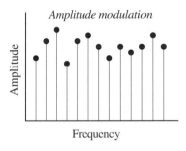

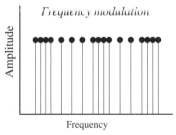

Information from mechanoreceptors to the CNS is conveyed by modulation of frequency and not by amplitude of the signal

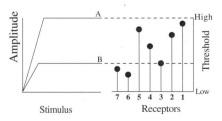

Stimulus B will only stimulate low-threshold receptors 3, 6 and 7. Stimulus A will activate all receptors

Figure 8.6 Frequency modulation and threshold.

mation in a joint will reduce the threshold levels of type III joint receptors, i.e. they become more sensitive to weak mechanical stimuli.[50] Sensitivity can also change at spinal cord level (see below).

Slow- and fast-adapting receptors

In response to a mechanical stimulus, the fast-adapting receptor will give a brief burst of activity, whereas the slow-adapting receptor will respond with a long decay period after the initial burst (Fig. 8.7). Some receptors are non-adapting and will continuously convey information as long as they are stimulated. For example, type IV joint nociceptors (pain receptors) do not adapt to mechanical stimuli.[50] The implication of this is discussed in Chapter 12.

Dynamic and static behaviour

Dynamic receptors are activated by movement (Fig. 8.7) and are often fast-adapting. Static receptors tend to have a steady-state firing rate even in stationary events, and are often slow-adapting. Generally speaking, dynamic receptors provide information about changes in limb position, whilst static receptors provide more continuous information about the position of the body in space. For example, moving the arm to rest it on a table activates both dynamic and static receptors. Once the arm is resting on the table, the dynamic receptors will fall silent. However, one is still aware of the position of the arm on the table from information conveyed by the static receptors.

GROUPS OF MECHANORECEPTORS

Practically speaking, mechanoreceptors can be divided into three broad anatomical groups:

1. muscle/tendon mechanoreceptors
2. joint mechanoreceptors
3. cutaneous mechanoreceptors.

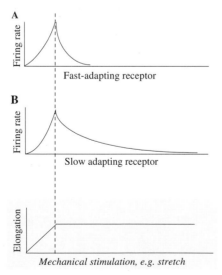
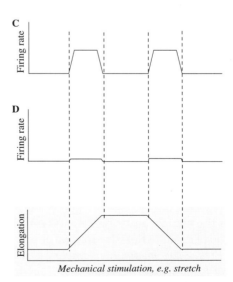

Figure 8.7 Functional properties of mechanoreceptors. (A) Fast-adapting receptors give a short burst of activity in response to a mechanical stimulus. (B) Slow-adapting receptors continue to fire for a period after the cessation of mechanical stimulation. (C) Dynamic receptors increase their firing rate during dynamic events but may be silent or have a low firing rate during static events. (D) Static receptors have a steady firing rate that may change little during dynamic events.

MUSCLE/TENDON MECHANORECEPTORS

There are two types of mechanoreceptor within the muscle–tendon unit: the muscle spindle, which is embedded within the muscle tissue itself and the Golgi tendon organ, situated within the tendon. In essence, both receptors work together to monitor various aspects of muscle activity and relay this information to the motor system (Fig. 8.8). In some muscles, the capsule of the spindle is fused or continues to form the capsule of the tendon organ. The anatomical proximity of the two receptors reflects their close functional relationship.[51]

Muscle spindles

Unlike other mechanoreceptors in the body, the muscle spindle contains contractile intrafusal fibres and sensory elements. Motor activation of the intrafusal fibres leads to changes in their tension and length, a variable calibration mechanism unique to the spindle. Such variability is essential for detecting the complex mechanical behaviour of the muscle.

Each muscle has a varying number of spindles depending on the intricacy of its performance. The more refined the function of the muscle, the greater the number of spindles per unit weight of the muscle. There are two groups

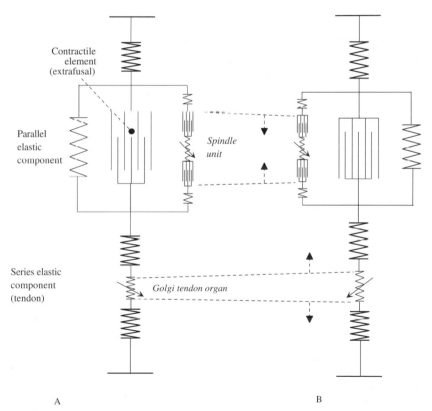

Figure 8.8 The muscle spindle and Golgi tendon organ provide information about mechanical events in the muscle–tendon unit. (A) The spindle units lie in parallel to the extrafusal muscle fibres, whereas the Golgi tendon organs lie in series with them. (B) During muscle contraction, the Golgi tendon organ conveys information about the force of contraction, whilst the muscle spindle conveys information about muscle length and changes in velocity.

of spindle afferents: primary endings (Ia) and secondary endings (II). Anatomically, the secondary afferents are situated at both sides of the primary afferent, but on average there is only one secondary to one primary as some spindles contain only primary afferents (Fig. 8.9). There are also other receptors within the muscle that are not related to detection of mechanical events. Functionally, spindle afferents convey information about different mechanical states of the muscle, such as length, velocity, acceleration, deceleration and, possibly to a lesser extent, force of contraction.[52,53] Their poor detection of contraction force is related to their anatomical position, lying in parallel to the extrafusal fibres within the connective tissue element of the muscle (see Fig. 8.8 above).

The primary spindle afferents are dynamic, fast-adapting receptors. They respond to changes of muscle length, velocity, acceleration and deceleration, and to muscle contraction. The secondary afferents are static, slow-adapting receptors that convey information about the instantaneous value of muscle length. The secon-

daries respond minimally to the velocity and force of contraction.[53]

Spindle stimulation by manipulation

Active and passive techniques. Probably the most important difference between active and passive techniques is the coactivation of intrafusal and extrafusal fibres during muscle contraction. During muscle contraction there is simultaneous motor drive to both the intrafusal and extrafusal fibres of the muscle.[54,55] The increase in motor drive to the intrafusal fibres tends to increase the spindle's firing rate and is closely graded with the force of contraction. This activity occurs in spite of the mechanical shortening of the muscle brought on by contraction. In fast movement against a light load, the spindle discharge tends to decrease transiently, but it is seldom totally abolished as may be the case during passive shortening of the muscle. If the contracting muscle is stretched, the overall firing rate will increase and follow the pattern of external loading. During high-force contractions,

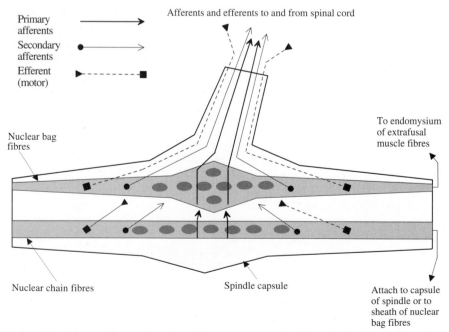

Figure 8.9 Schematic representation of the muscle spindle (After Gray's 1980 with permission from Churchill Livingstone.[235])

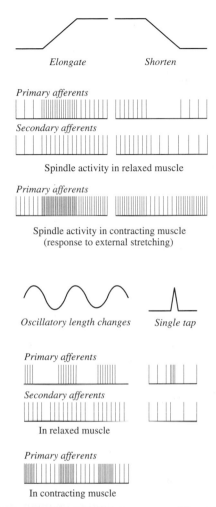

Figure 8.10 Spindle activity in response to different forms of external loading. (After Matthews 1964 with permission from the American Physiological Society.[58])

external loading has less influence over the firing rate of the spindle (Fig. 8.10).[56]

In relaxed muscle, the primary and secondary endings generally have a low firing rate, some being silent at medium muscle length (which corresponds to the resting position of the joint).[26] In this position, fewer than 10% of the spindle primaries are discharging.[59] This low rate of discharge is related to the quiescence of fusimotor drive.[55,60] This prominent difference in firing rate between active and passive states indicates the reduced ability of the spindle to measure muscle length in the passive state (see below).[26,59]

During sinusoidal stretching of a relaxed or

contracting muscle, the primary afferent fires during the lengthening phase and falls silent during shortening. However, during contraction, the overall firing rate is much higher in comparison with that occurring in passive oscillation of the muscle.[61] As the force of contraction increases, the spindle will also fire during the shortening phase of the oscillation (Fig. 8.10).[57]

Dynamic and static techniques. The spindle afferents have a higher firing rate during dynamic than static events (Fig. 8.10). During muscle stretching, the overall firing rate increases. Once the stretch is completed and the muscle is held in its lengthened position, the overall activity of the spindle decreases. If the muscle is passively shortened, the firing rate of the primary afferent is markedly slowed. This change in the firing pattern may provide important feedback information and is probably very different from spindle silence when the muscle is held passively in its resting position.

The rate (velocity) of stretching also alters the firing rate of the spindle primaries: increased velocity of stretching tends to increase their overall firing rate. This response occurs in both active and passive manipulation. The spindle primaries are very sensitive to extremely small changes in the muscle length. They have been shown to be a hundred-fold more sensitive to low-amplitude than high-amplitude stretches.[52]

Manual implications. The size of discharge from the spindle afferent can be influenced by the mode of manipulation. A large barrage of information from the spindle can be induced by dynamic rather than sustained stretches. Further increased activity can be generated by active–dynamic techniques (Fig. 8.11).

Golgi tendon organs

Golgi tendon organs are situated within the tendon fascicle close to the musculotendinous junction. They are connected to 10–20 muscle fibres and are not affected by mechanical events in other muscle fibres. However, they can be unloaded by the contraction of neighbouring fibres.

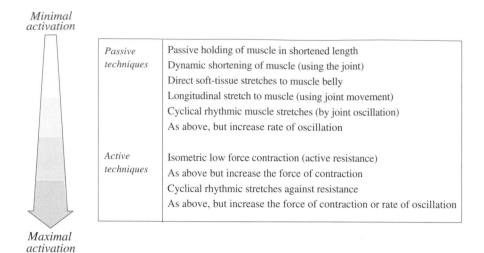

Minimal activation

Passive techniques	Passive holding of muscle in shortened length
	Dynamic shortening of muscle (using the joint)
	Direct soft-tissue stretches to muscle belly
	Longitudinal stretch to muscle (using joint movement)
	Cyclical rhythmic muscle stretches (by joint oscillation)
	As above, but increase rate of oscillation
Active techniques	Isometric low force contraction (active resistance)
	As above but increase the force of contraction
	Cyclical rhythmic stretches against resistance
	As above, but increase the force of contraction or rate of oscillation

Maximal activation

Figure 8.11 Summary of how spindle activity may be maximized or minimized by manipulation.

The Golgi tendon organs convey information about the force of muscle contraction.[51,52] They are not stretch receptors as is sometimes believed. They are so sensitive to the force of contraction (low threshold) that contraction of a single muscle fibre to which they are attached will bring about an increase in their discharge.

Golgi stimulation by manipulation

Active versus passive technique. It has been demonstrated that the tendon organ is more sensitive to active (muscle contraction) than passive (passive stretch) force. This insensitivity to passive stretches is due to the anatomical location of the receptor within the muscle–tendon unit. The tendon organ lies in series with the fascicle of the muscle fibres and in parallel to most of the connective tissue within and around the muscle (Fig. 8.12A). During passive stretches, the parallel elastic component (the belly of the muscle) accounts for much of the muscle's passive elongation, because the parallel is less stiff than the series elastic component. The tendon organ, which lies in series, is therefore only weakly affected by stretching (Fig. 8.12B).[51] This is further supported by studies demonstrating that a passive stretch of the cat soleus muscle producing 500 g in the whole tendon

will exert no more than 50 mg force on a single Golgi fascicle. This is lower than the force produced by a single contracting muscle fibre.[52]

Dynamic versus static technique. The relationship between the force of contraction and the firing rate of the Golgi tendon organ is nonlinear, except in low-force contractions; i.e. an increase in the force of contraction does not produce a proportional increase in the Golgi organ's firing rate. It has been suggested that the Golgi tendon organ's main role is to provide information about dynamic changes in force during muscle contraction.[51] This implies that dynamic rather than static muscle contractions will have a greater effect on the Golgi organ's firing rate.

Manual implication. Passive stretching of muscle is ineffective at stimulating Golgi tendon organs. Active techniques will stimulate them to a greater extent, active dynamic techniques being more effective than active static (isometric) ones.

JOINT RECEPTORS

Through their overall contribution to proprioception, joint afferents play an important role in the overall functional stability of joints.[62–64] Joint mechanoreceptors detect mechanical changes at the joint and convey information

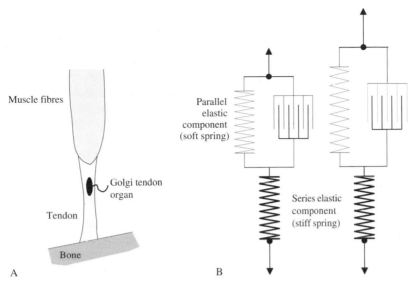

Muscle fibres

Golgi tendon organ

Tendon

Bone

A

Parallel
elastic
component
(soft spring)

Series elastic
component
(stiff spring)

B

Figure 8.12   The Golgi tendon organ lies in the series elastic component (tendon of muscle), which is stiffer than the parallel elastic component (epimysium, perimysium and endomysium). During passive stretches of the muscle, the parallel elastic component will elongate to a greater extent than the series elastic component.

about the range, speed and position of the joint to the motor system. Their role in proprioception can be clearly seen when the joint afferents are anaesthetized.[65] In such circumstances, the ability of the subject to judge the position of the joint during passive movement is greatly reduced. When only part of the capsule is anaesthetized, proprioception in one direction is preferentially affected. For example, when the dorsal aspect of the big toe is anaesthetized, proprioceptive acuity is reduced in passive flexion but is unimpaired in extension.

Joint receptors respond to different modes (active/passive) of joint loading as well as to the pattern of loading (rate, direction and range). Most joint afferents are only responsive to a movement arc of about 15– 20°. As the movement of the joint enters the receptor's range, it will increase its firing rate. When the movement exceeds its range, it will reduce its firing rate or become totally silent.[4]

Most synovial joints have four types of receptors. Groups I, II and III are stimulated by changes of tension in the tissue in which they are embedded. Group IV receptors are pain receptors and are usually active following joint injury.[50]

Group I mechanoreceptors

These are embedded in the outer fibrous part of the joint capsule. They are low-threshold receptors that respond to very small changes in the tension of the capsule. Some units are of such low threshold that they fire continuously even when the joint is not moving. These receptors are slow adapting, and their frequency of resting discharge rises and falls in proportion to increases and decreases in the tension of the capsule. They are different from fast-adapting receptors, which generally give out a short burst of activity in response to alterations in tension. Abnormal movement beyond the joint's physiological range will also increase their firing rate. Their low-threshold characteristics mean that they can be stimulated even by applying direct pressure to the joint capsule or ligaments.[66,67] However, rubbing the capsule of the knee joint will not give rise to a sensation of joint movement.

Group I receptors are both dynamic and static receptors; i.e. they continuously convey positional information in the immobile joint, whilst in the mobile joint they signal the direction, amplitude and velocity of movement.[68]

Group II mechanoreceptors

These are also embedded in the fibrous aspect of the capsule, but deeper and closer to the synovial tissue.[50] They are rapidly adapting dynamic mechanoreceptors, inactive in immobile joints and active in moving ones. They give a short burst of impulses when the tension in the capsule rises, for example when the joint is stretched or articulated.[68]

Group III mechanoreceptors

These are dynamic, high-threshold receptors that become active during abnormal mechanical stresses at extreme joint positions or in pathological joint conditions where there is effusion or inflammation. These receptors become sensitized during inflammation and their threshold decreases.[69] This sensitivity is mediated locally at the receptor site by inflammatory byproducts. There is also neurological sensitization occuring at spinal cord level, which will be discussed below.[70]

Group IV nociceptors

These are high-threshold pain receptors that are active during joint inflammation, effusion and extreme mechanical stress. Although they are not true mechanoreceptors, some are activated by movement, albeit providing a poor sense of joint position.[70]

Joint afferent stimulation by manipulation

Dynamic versus static, and active versus passive technique

Movement, whether active or passive, will stimulate the joint's dynamic receptors (groups I and II mechanoreceptors). Overall, dynamic techniques will recruit a larger number of afferent groups and increase their firing rate. In some joints, such as the knee, where the tendon invades the joint capsule, contraction of the muscle can increase the tension, in the capsule, leading to increased joint afferent activity.[16,60] The recruitment of the different joint afferents during static and dynamic techniques is summarized in Fig. 8.13.

SKIN MECHANORECEPTORS

The role of skin afferents in proprioception is to provide information about sensory events, for example when contact with a surface is made during a reaching movement, and surface textures.[71] Skin afferents also contribute to fast reflexive gripping when an object is slipping through the hand and play a role in providing information on joint movement. These sensations arise when the skin over the joint is stretched by movement, as has been demonstrated by microstimulation of skin mechanoreceptors near the nailbed, which elicits a sensation of flexion at the distal interphalangeal joint.[72] This illusion is consistent with the receptor's signal pattern when the joint is passively flexed. Proprioception has also been shown to be enhanced by applying an elasticated bandage around a damaged joints: the feedback from the skin complements the reduced proprioception from the joint receptors.

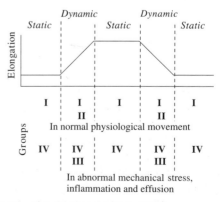

Figure 8.13 Functional properties of joint mechanoreceptors.

Essentially, there are four types of skin mechanoreceptors: two fast-adapting (dynamic RA and PC receptors) and two slow-adapting (SA1 and SA2 static) receptors.[73]

Manual stimulation of skin mechanoreceptors

Active versus passive technique

There is no great difference between active and passive techniques in stimulating the skin afferents.

Dynamic versus static technique

Dynamic responses predominate over static responses when the skin is deformed by external forces. For example, vigorous discharges are induced by vibration of the skin, by an indentation moving along the skin surface and by rapid intermittent pressure of the skin. In comparison, sustained indentation produces only moderate static activity.[26,54] Some receptors are highly sensitive and will respond to skin stretches and light taps several centimetres from the centre of their field of reception.

The relatively higher sensitivity of skin mechanoreceptors to dynamic stimuli can be demonstrated by comparing a constant pressure with a finger on the skin to the sensation of continuously rubbing the skin. During static pressure, there is rapid adaptation and within a very short period the compressed skin will almost feel numb. In contrast, the sensation and awareness of the hand moving across the skin will be felt throughout the time the skin is rubbed.

The ability to distinguish between different surface textures is higher when the skin brushes against the surface than in the absence of such movement.[54] This can be felt by touching different surfaces with the eyes shut. To begin with, hold a finger on each surface without moving it; then repeat the same procedure, but now gently brush the finger against the surface. During sustained touch, it is virtually impossible to perceive surface textures. Movement of the skin against the surface markedly improves the ability to differentiate between textures.

SUMMARY: AFFERENT RECRUITMENT BY MANIPULATION

The proprioceptive barrage to the motor system will vary according to the mode and pattern of the manual event. For example, during massage, predominantly skin afferents are recruited, with some increase in spindle firing rate (as a result of stretches of the underlying muscle fibres). In articulation, joint afferents are activated, together with the spindle afferents of the muscles acting over the joint. The effect of the modes of technique on different receptors is outlined in Table 8.1.

Size and pattern of afferent feedback

The size or magnitude of the afferent discharge can be modified by different techniques. Changes in its magnitude can be generated by two mechanisms (Fig. 8.14):

- temporal volley
- spatial volley.

Temporal volley

Temporal volley is used to describe the increase in firing rate of the same group of receptors. For example, joints afferents can be made to increase their firing rate by increasing the velocity of stretching. A temporal increase in spindle discharge can be achieved by increasing the force of contraction or by increasing the rate of muscle stretching.

The importance of temporal volley in position detection has been demonstrated in skin, joints and muscle receptors. Direct stimulation of single afferents by microelectrodes usually (but not always) fails to arouse perception of movement.[72] The perception of movement arises only when a sufficient number of the same receptors are stimulated. A further example of temporal volley is demonstrated in passive joint movement. The awareness of joint position is

Table 8.1 Receptor recruitment during different modes of manual technique

Receptor type	Functional behaviour	Manual techniques			
		Passive–static	Passive–dynamic	Active–static	Active–dynamic
Spindle primary	Static and dynamic Respond to changes in muscle length, velocity and force of contraction	Active	More active	Attenuated sensitivity and activity	Highly active
Spindle secondary	Static receptors Respond to changes in muscle length	Active	Active but less than type 1a afferent	As primaries but less sensitive	Highly active but less sensitive
Golgi tendon organ	Respond to changes in the force of muscle contraction	Inactive	Inactive	Active	Very active
Articular I	Static and dynamic Low threshold Slow adapting Active in immobile and mobile joints	Active	More active	Active	More active
Articular II	Dynamic Low threshold Fast adapting Respond to joint movement	Inactive	Active	Inactive	Active
Articular III	Dynamic High threshold Active in extreme joint position, inflammation and effusion	Inactive	Active (see text)	Inactive	Active (see text)
Skin mechano-receptors	Fast-adapting dynamic Slow-adapting static Respond to skin stretches, indentation, rubbing and vibration	Active	Active if joint movement is coupled with movement of hands on the skin	Active only if associated with movement of hands on the skin	Active only if associated with movement of hands on the

markedly increased during rapid passive motion,[72] whereas slow passive motion contributes very little to the perception of joint position. Although the same group of afferents is being activated, the overall afferent volley is increased in the rapid movement mode, corresponding to increased proprioceptive acuity by the subjects. Similarly, when active and mildly resisted movements are used to assess proprioceptive acuity in leg positioning, acuity tends to rise in the resisted mode.[74] This rise in acuity is probably related to an increase in the temporal activity of muscle receptors as the force of contraction increases.

Spatial volley

Spatial volley is related to the simultaneous activation of several receptor groups. For example, in active–dynamic techniques, there is spatial activation of muscle and joint afferents.

The importance of spatial volley can be demonstrated when a subject is tested for acuity during active–static and active–dynamic finger movement.[75] Acuity rises during dynamic finger movements and falls with static modes. In these two modes, different groups of afferents are being activated. In the active–static mode, muscle secondary afferents and Golgi afferents are activated with some activation of the muscle primaries. In the active–dynamic mode, afferent activity from the muscle primaries and joint receptors is the total afferent volley. The increase in diversity of the receptors corresponds to an increased awareness of joint position. In this example, the increased volley is due not solely to augmented spatial volley, but also to the increased temporal activity from

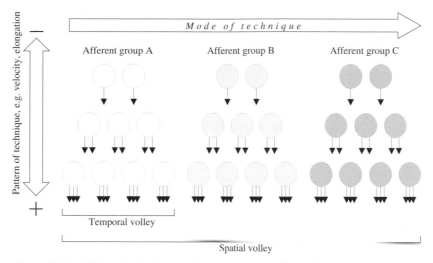

Figure 8.14 Different technique modes and patterns will alter the volume of the afferent volley. Different groups of receptors are represented by different shading. Increased temporal activity can arise by an increased firing rate of single receptors as well as by recruitment of a larger number of receptors (within the same group of mechanoreceptors). Velocity, elongation of tissues and force of contraction will largely affect temporal volley. Spatial volley will be influenced by the mode of technique, i.e. active, passive, dynamic or static.

the Golgi tendon organs and the spindle afferents.

A combination of spatial and temporal volleys probably reflects the true afferent activity during normal motor activity. Feedback about movement converges on the motor system from a wide array of receptors (joint, skin and muscle afferents). An important principle is that single groups of receptors cannot be singled out during manipulation: any manual technique will involve a varying number of these. The belief that some forms of technique will only stimulate the Golgi tendon body or the spindle afferents cannot be maintained. However, manipulation may have some capacity to modulate the overall temporal and spatial activity (Fig. 8.14).

LOWER MOTOR SYSTEM RESPONSE TO MANIPULATION

SUBORGANIZATION OF THE MOTOR SYSTEM

There is some evidence for a functional sub-organization of the different motor centres within the total motor system, i.e. a subunit of executive, efferent and sensory feedback within the macroorganization (see Fig. 8.1 above). This organization is sometimes referred to as the lower motor system. This suborganization can also be demonstrated in the spinal cord.[76] Animals that have had their spinal cord severed at the level of T12 can be trained to generate almost normal walking with the hindlimb when placed on a treadmill.[77] Such an animal is capable of quite remarkable processing of afferent information in the absence of higher centres. When the skin of the paw is stimulated during the swing phase, the whole limb reflexly flexes to evade an obstacle and then proceeds with walking. In similar experimental conditions, the animal will use the hindlimb for scratching if a flea moves on its fur.[78] This suggests that, within the spinal cord, there is an executive, an efferent and a sensory feedback system that is capable of producing complex motor acts in virtual autonomy from the rest of the motor system. However, this lower motor system is primitive in function and is unable to produce the complex movement patterns of the whole system. This suborganization is probably involved in fast adjustments during movement. Placed anatomically and functionally lower within the motor system, and with short reflex loops, this organization is well placed for providing such rapid responses. The existence of such a suborganization may be related to evolution in mammals, where more recent higher centres have developed over ancient spinal centres. The old spinal centres, however, did not become redundant but were integrated into the evolving nervous system.[53]

In the intact motor system, the lower motor system is under the dominant influence of the higher motor centres. Some neurons in the cortex have a direct monosynaptic connection with the spinal motorneurons (interestingly the bulk of this corticomotorneural pathway is largest in man in comparison with other primates).[79] In central nervous system damage, the control of the higher over the lower motor system may be lost, leading to spontaneous, non-purposeful motor activity from the spinal centres.

General considerations

One commonly held belief in manual therapy is that the lower motor system can be influenced by manipulation. Because the lower motor system represents the final motor pathway to the muscle, it is assumed that stimulating different mechanoreceptors by manipulation will alter the activity of this organization and motor tone to the muscles.

Afferent fibres from mechanoreceptors converge segmentally on the dorsal horn of the spinal cord (Fig. 8.15). Once within the spinal cord, this segmental anatomy is somewhat lost. The fibres tend to diverge in an ascending and descending manner, over several segments, synapsing with different neuronal pools and spinal interneurons. This has functional logic as normal activity involves total body movement occurring over many joints and muscle groups. The information about activity in one group of muscles has to be conveyed to all other muscles taking part in the movement. Flexing

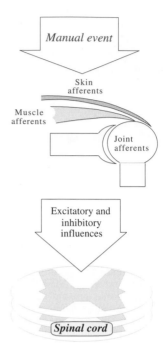

Figure 8.15 Afferents communicate with the central aspect of the motor system via inhibition or excitation. Note that these influences are feedback and cannot control the motor drive from the higher centres.

the knee, for example, involves activity of the hip muscles and lower back, as well as other postural adjustments.

The motorneurons of several muscles are intermingled in any region of the motorneuron cell column and many synergistic group of muscles share common afferent inputs.[80] This means that spindle afferents from one group of muscles supply not only the motorneurons of the muscle in which they are embedded, but also other synergistic muscles. This implies that any attempt to perform neuromanipulation of a single segment can be totally abandoned: even the most specific and localized form of manipulation will be transmitted to a broad anatomical and functional area within the nervous system.

The motorneurons are subject to inhibitory and excitatory influences, primarily from descending ones from the higher centres and to a lesser extent from peripheral influences arising in different mechanoreceptors. Descending motor pathways converge largely on spinal interneurons and to a lesser extent directly on motor-neurons. The dendritic surface area (the receptive area) of each motorneuron is quite extensive, taking up approximately 97% of the total surface area of the cell. This highlights the extent of inputs to the motorneuron.[80] Peripheral information arriving at the spinal cord generally affects the motorneurons of both agonist and antagonist muscles (Fig. 8.16). In some instances, these influences may be opposing; for example, if an afferent source inhibits the agonists, it may also have excitatory influences on the antagonists, and vice versa. Such opposing activations, arising from different receptors embedded within the same muscle, probably act in a fashion similar to that of central inhibitory and excitatory influences; together they act as feedback to refine the motor output.[81]

It should be noted that *the influences that proprioceptors have on the motorneuron pool are very mild in comparison with those of descending influences from the higher centres.* Furthermore, all the reflexive influences that proprioceptors have on motorneurons are task dependent (see below). We will now consider the reflex influences of mechanoreceptors on motorneurons. These influences are only valid for the particular condition of each study, for example the position of the limb and the type of background motor activity, and the reflex response in one situation cannot be inferred to all other limb positions or movements.

SEGMENTAL INFLUENCES OF SPINDLE AFFERENTS

Although the spindle afferents are the best

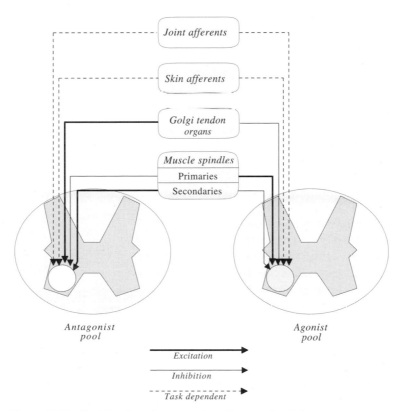

Figure 8.16   Peripheral mechanoreceptor influences (excitation and inhibition) on agonist and antagonist motorneuron pools. Note that these represent the overall influence of the afferent groups. Some of these influences are transmitted to the motorneuron via interneurons or by the effects of one group of afferents on another via spinal interneurons.

documented of the peripheral mechanoreceptors, they should not be thought of as having the most important input to the motorneuron pool. The spindle primaries contribute only about 1% to the ensemble of inputs to the motorneuron.[80]

The spindle primary and secondary afferents have been shown to have opposing influences on the motorneurons (Fig. 8.16). Primary spindle afferents have an overall excitatory effect on the agonistic motorneuron and an inhibitory influence on the antagonistic motorneurons (reciprocal inhibition).[31,82] The spindle secondaries have an inhibitory influence on the agonist motorneuron pool and possibly an excitatory influence on the antagonist pool. This seemingly opposite effect of the primaries and secondaries does not act to switch the motorneurons on and off, but contributes to the formation of the sensory feedback map.

The influence of the primary afferents on motor activity is often demonstrated by the tonic vibration reflex.[83] When a high-frequency vibration is applied to the tendon or muscle belly, it excites the primary spindle afferents, producing a reflex contraction of the agonist muscle with a simultaneous relaxation of the antagonistic muscle.[82] The tonic vibratory reflex is used clinically to induce an inhibitory state in muscles that are under increased neurological tone (such as in spasticity).[84–87] In this situation, the vibrator is applied to the flaccid antagonist muscle to produce inhibition of the overactive agonist muscle. Here, *peripheral inhibition is replacing lost central control* (which may be lost inhibition or increased excitation). However, this inhibitory response is very mild in comparison with descending, central inhibitory control and therefore cannot replace central inhibition. Furthermore, the motor system may habituate to the repeated peripheral stimulation, leading to a progressively decreasing response.

Another more common example of the role of spindle afferents is the tendon reflex. It is widely accepted that the most important afferents in this reflex are the spindle primaries, which are sensitive to the sudden length changes in the muscle induced by a brisk tap.[31]

Manual implications

It has long been believed that manual techniques such as high-velocity thrusts or adjustments can normalize abnormal motor tone. The reduced motor tone is attributed to the stimulation of inhibitory afferents by manipulation. This is highly unlikely as sudden stretch produced by this form of manipulation will excite rather than inhibit the motorneuron.

SEGMENTAL INFLUENCES OF THE GOLGI TENDON ORGAN

Golgi afferents have inhibitory influences on the agonist motorneuron (autogenic inhibition) and excitatory ones on the antagonist motorneuron pool (Fig. 8.16).[81] These influences do not act as on–off switches for the motorneuron, otherwise the excitatory influence of the primaries and the inhibitory influence of the Golgi tendon organ would cancel each other out.

In neurologically healthy individuals, the Golgi tendon organ has a very mild reflexogenic effect on the motorneuron pool. Hence, manual techniques that claim to influence this group of afferents will be ineffective when treating neurologically healthy individuals. The reflexogenic effect of the Golgi tendon organs only becomes stronger and more apparent in pathological states of the nervous system, such as in certain forms of upper motor lesion. For example, the clasp-knife reflex, which is attributed to the inhibitory influences of the Golgi tendon organ on its own muscle (other muscle afferents are probably also involved in this reflex).[51,53]

SEGMENTAL INFLUENCES OF SKIN AFFERENTS

The pattern of inhibition and excitation produced by skin mechanoreceptors seems to be highly variable, depending on the form of stimulation and the ongoing motor activity (i.e. it is task dependent). In relaxed individuals, stimulation of the skin afferents in the leg has an overall inhibitory influence on the motorneurons supplying the leg muscles.[88] Stimulation of the skin during movement and muscle contraction presents a more complex mixture of inhibitory and excitatory influences. The response tends to spread to the motorneuron pools of the whole limb and even the contralateral limb.[89] Excitatory responses to skin stimulation can be seen when the sole of the foot is scratched and the toes curl downwards (the Babinski reflex), in the cremasteric reflex as the testicles ascend in response to stroking the inner thigh, and the abdominal muscle contraction in response to scratching the abdominal skin.

SEGMENTAL INFLUENCES OF JOINT AFFERENTS

The joint receptors tend to contribute to the ensemble of sensory inputs converging on the motorneurons supplying the intrafusal (spindle) fibres rather than directly influencing the extra-fusal motorneurons (Fig. 8.17).[62,64,90–93]

There is much controversy over the contribution of joint afferents to the inhibition or excitation processes of the extrafusal motorneuron

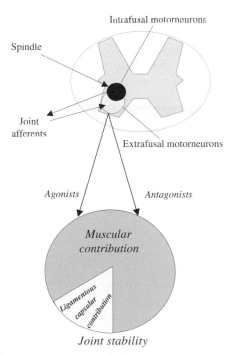

Figure 8.17 Schematic representation of joint afferent influences on the spinal cord and their contribution to joint stability during activity.

pool. The overall consensus is that *in healthy joints their reflex effect is very low*, but some reflex excitation of the antagonist motorneuron pool may take place when the joint is maximally stretched; i.e. full forceful extension of the knee may produce excitation of the hamstring motorneuron pool. Flexion of the knee seems to reverse that pattern, leading to inhibition of the hamstrings.[94] Similar to the situation with other proprioceptors, the reflex response is confined not only to pathways of the hip muscles, but also to pathways of the knee and ankle muscles.[95] The potency of the joint afferents in influencing motor processes rises only when there is joint damage. This reflexogenic influence is discussed in more detail in Chapter 10.

TASK-DEPENDENT REFLEXES

Peripherally mediated reflexes are heavily modulated by central motor processes (descending motor activity from higher centres).[96] It has been shown that the response to the stretch reflex can be routed to an antagonist muscle group if it is advantageous to the movement.[28] The original state of the animal limb is also important and will modulate the response in favour of the ongoing programme. For example, if the cutaneous afferents of the paw of a walking cat are stimulated during the swing phase (as the limb is moving into flexion), it will reinforce the flexion movement. If the same stimulus is applied when the limb is moving into extension, it will reinforce extension of the limb.[77] Similarly, stimulation of human cutaneous afferents in the leg results in short- and long-latency reflexes, which can be either inhibitory or excitatory in relation to the current posture or activity.[89] In much the same way, the gain of the stretch reflex is modulated during the walking cycle by central motor centres.[97] If the quadriceps stretch reflex is elicited while the limb is moving into extension, the reflex amplitude of the EMG will rise. Conversely, when the limb is moving into flexion, the quadriceps stretch reflex may be inhibited.

The reflex response is not simply dependent on ongoing motor activity: other proprioceptive inputs may also alter it. For example, joint afferents have been shown to influence transmission within the Golgi tendon organ pathway.[98] This is not limited to joint afferents, as other groups of receptors also have the ability to influence each other's transmission.

These studies highlight a very important principle in the motor control of movement: that descending motor drives, which dominate movement production, can override or totally eliminate peripherally mediated activity. Proprioceptors have only a mild reflexive influence on moment-to-moment motor activity, so manual techniques that rely on proprioceptive reflexes will have only a mild effect on the motor system, or none at all. Another important principle is that motor activity is so extensive and complex, with intertwined components, that it cannot be fragmented and observed. All one can see is general, overall patterns. Techniques that rely on single reflexes cannot predict the enormity and complexity within which these reflexes have to work. These principles will be explored from different perspectives throughout this section.

MANUAL INFLUENCES ON THE LOWER MOTOR SYSTEM AND MOTORNEURON EXCITABILITY

Studies have recently been conducted to assess the influence of different manual techniques on motorneuron excitability. These studies consider whether the stimulation of proprioceptors by manipulation can reflexively affect the activity of the motorneuron pool; i.e. if a muscle is neurologically overactive, can manipulation inhibit that muscle's motorneurons?

To test the excitability of motorneurons, the spindle afferents are stimulated by different methods, for example tendon tap, sudden stretch or electrical stimulation of the receptor's axon. This stimulation results in excitation of the muscle's motorneuron pool, with a consequent reflex muscle contraction, the force of which is expressed as a change in amplitude of the EMG signal or a change of force as recorded by a strain gauge. This serves as an indirect method of assessing motorneuron excitability: the more excitable the motorneuron, the higher the force of contraction and the EMG amplitude. In inhibition, the opposite happens, with reduced EMG amplitude.

EFFECT OF MANUAL TECHNIQUES ON MOTORNEURON EXCITABILITY IN NEUROLOGICALLY HEALTHY SUBJECTS

Continuous and intermittent manual pressure on tendons

Continuous and intermittent manual pressure on tendons has been shown to decrease motorneuron excitability. This inhibitory influence was present in normal individuals as well as in patients with stroke.[99,100] The effect of intermittent pressure was greater than that of continuous pressure. The manual pressures used in these studies were approximately 5 kg and 10 kg, and no significant differences were found between these two loading levels. It is likely that the inhibition observed in these studies was related to the activation of cutaneous afferents rather than muscle receptors. Muscle receptors can be activated by tapping;[26] however, one would expect that stimulation of the spindle afferents would increase the excitability of motorneurons rather than leading to the inhibition observed. Golgi afferents are unlikely to be the source of inhibition as the manual pressure is not high enough to stimulate them. To stimulate the Golgi by a passive technique, one would need to apply a much greater force in a stretching pattern rather than in compression (see below). The fact that intermittent compression had a greater inhibitory influence also implicates cutaneous receptors that are markedly more active during dynamic stimuli. A further surprising finding was that the tapping induced a state of inhibition in patients displaying spasticity. These findings are contradicted by studies showing increased excitability during stretch and vibration in patients with upper motorneuron lesions;[101] one would expect similar results (exaggerated excitation) when tapping the tendons of patients suffering from spasticity.

Manual tapping of muscle belly

Reduced motorneuron excitability has also been observed during a study of manual tapping of the muscle belly,[102] using a rate of 4 Hz for a period of 30 seconds. In this study, the excitability of the soleus motorneurons was recorded in response to tapping of the receptor-bearing muscle, i.e. the soleus muscle as well as the ipsilateral hamstring and tibialis anterior. Tapping of all these different areas resulted in reduced soleus motorneuron excitability, regardless of the site of manual tapping. It implies that afferents other than muscle receptors were being activated by the tapping. One reason for this assumption was discussed above in regard to tendon tapping: it would be expected that the muscle primaries would be stimulated, resulting in excitatory rather than inhibitory influences. Furthermore, stimulation of synergist muscle afferents (the hamstring) would be expected to increase rather than depress excitability. It is possible that, in manual tapping, skin afferents overlying these muscles are being activated, skin afferents having been shown to produce widespread inhibitory influences throughout the limb.[89] It has also been shown that cutaneous stimulation, such as scratching of the limb, has an inhibitory influence on the soleus motorneurons of healthy subjects.[88]

Massage

Massage applied to the muscle belly has also been shown transiently to reduce motorneuron excitability.[103] Two intensities of massage were used in this study with the higher intensity massage producing greater inhibition.[104] Similar results of reduced motoneurone excitability have been observed in patients with spinal cord injury.[105]

Muscle stretching

The change in motorneuron excitability has been studied during three different forms of stretching commonly used in exercise and sports:[106] passive stretches of the muscle (soleus); maximal antago-

nist (pretibial muscle) contraction superimposed on stretching; and full voluntary contraction of the agonist muscle for 10 seconds superseded by passive stretches of the muscle. In all three forms of stretching, there was found to be reduced excitability of the motorneuron pool supplying the stretched muscle. This inhibitory effect was greater in the active modes of stretching, i.e. agonist contraction–relaxation and antagonist contraction. The greatest inhibitory state was produced by antagonist contraction. It is likely that this extra inhibition seen in active stretching is as a result of central inhibition, i.e. higher centres instructing one group of muscles to contract and its antagonist group to relax. Such activity is not present in relaxed stretched muscle, hence the difference in the inhibitory state between active and passive stretching. The inhibitory response in the passive mode of stretching may be mediated by the secondary spindle afferents from the soleus muscle itself. It is unlikely that this inhibition would arise from the stimulation of the Golgi afferents as they are not involved in passive stretches of the muscle. The inhibition recorded in the stretched muscle following agonist contraction was attributed to 'post-contraction inhibition,' whatever that may be. In all three modalities of stretching, the inhibitory state lasted only for the duration of the stretching, returning immediately to the prestretch levels.

Manual effleurage

Manual effleurage over the muscle has also been shown to reduce motorneuron excitability.[107]

The spinal influences of the different manual techniques are summarized in Table 8.2.

Effects of active, passive, dynamic and static manual techniques

In all the above studies, the pretest and posttest measurements were carried out with the patient fully relaxed. This means that the effect of manipulation is not assessed against an ongoing

Table 8.2 Changes in motorneuron excitability following different manual techniques: the only technique to have a carry-over effect following the cessation of manipulation was the active–dynamic technique (shaded row)

Manual technique	Description of technique	Motorneuron excitability	Excitability changes during manipulation	Excitability carry-over following manipulation
Stretch reflex tested while subjects fully relaxed				
Continuous and intermittent pressure on tendon	Two pressures used; 10 kg and 5 kg Subject passive	Inhibition	Yes	No
Manual tapping of muscle belly	Frequency of tapping 4 Hz for 30 s Subject passive	Inhibition	Yes	No
Massage	For 3 min Subject passive	Inhibition	Yes	No
Effleurage	Over distance of 20–25 cm Subject passive	Inhibition	Yes	No
1. Passive muscle stretching	Soleus stretch by foot dorsiflexion for 25 s Subject passive	Inhibition	Yes Lasting 10 s	No
2. Passive muscle stretching	Preceded by 10 s of agonists 100% MVC	Inhibition	Yes	No
3. Passive muscle stretching	Agonist contraction while antagonists being stretched (calf muscle)	Inhibition	Yes	No
Stretch reflex tested while subjects maintained 10% MVC				
Massage directly to muscle	For period of 5 min			No
Joint articulation	Knee flexion oscillation for 5 min Approx. 700 cycles in total			No
Isometric contraction	Isometric contraction at 50% MVC 8 repetitions lasting 10 s			No
Knee and hip extension against resistance	8 × 10 s cycles of knee and hip extension against resistance	Inhibition		Yes Lasting up to 55 s

MVC, Maximal voluntary contraction.

voluntary contraction to see whether the motor system has 'acknowledged' the change, or whether the change can survive a motor event initiated by higher centres. After all, any change achieved by treatment should survive volitional activity and in some way affect it. The effects of manipulation on the stretch reflex during volutary activation have been examined in our own studies. Four modalities of manual technique were tested: soft-tissue massage to the quadriceps muscle (passive–static), knee oscillation at 90° (passive–dynamic), eight cycles of isometric contractions (active–static) and eight cycles of active hip and knee extension (active–dynamic). Of these, only the active–dynamic

techniques made a significant change to the amplitude of the stretch reflex (Table 8.2), (D Newham & E Lederman, unpublished work, 1995) although this effect lasted for less than 1 minute. The results of this and the above studies question the ability of manipulation to alter motorneuron excitability by the stimulation of proprioceptors.

EFFECT OF MANUAL TECHNIQUES ON MOTORNEURON EXCITABILITY IN PATIENTS WITH CENTRAL NERVOUS DAMAGE

As with normal individuals, manual techniques

in patients with central nervous system pathologies appear to have no longlasting effect on the excitability of the motorneurons. In all of these studies, changes in excitability occurred only during manipulation. The techniques that have been tested are intermittent and continuous manual pressure on the tendon,[99,100] and massage.[105]

MANUAL LIMITATION IN CONTROLLING THE MOTOR SYSTEM FROM THE PERIPHERY

The influence of proprioceptors on the nervous system is minimal in comparison with that of motor drives from higher centres (Fig. 8.18).[3,20] There is a biological logic behind such arrangement. If the sensory system had dominant control over the motor system, it would mean that external events could disturb and overwhelm the integratory processes of the CNS. For example, during walking, stimulation of the skin afferents in the leg inhibits the motorneurons of the leg muscles. If these inhibitory

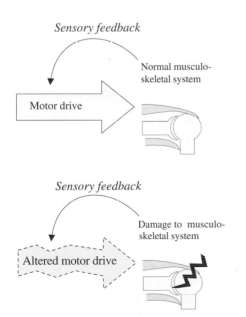

Figure 8.18   Central motor drive has a dominant control over motor events. The motor response may be more attentive to sensory influences when the information relayed has a protective meaning.

influences had a dominant influence over central motor activity, the friction produced by wearing trousers would result in the total disruption of walking. Similarly, if the skin of the arm were to rub against some surface while lifting a heavy box, it would result in inhibition of the arm motorneurons and a sudden loss of strength. Naturally, this event does not happen during physical activity. The inhibitory process is only a small part within the total schema of feedback and does not 'switch off' the motorneurons.

The stimulation of the proprioceptor results in weak reflex muscle contraction that has no functional role in movement; reflex contraction elicited by a tendon tap is minimal in comparison with background voluntary contraction. When tested in the presence of background muscular activity, the tendon reflex produces a small increase in force of about 3% above background force.[34] This reflex force generation is relatively constant in relation to varying levels of voluntary contraction. Much the same occurs in reciprocal inhibition: the force reduction in the antagonist muscle is about 2–4% below the background contraction level.[82]

This implies that the reflex responses initiated peripherally by manipulation will have only a relatively mild influence on the immediate activity of the *intact* CNS. Only in pathological situations, such as central damage to the motor system, does mechanoreceptor influence increase to disturb motor activity (Figs 8.18 and 8.19). In such circumstances, the influence of the different reflex mechanisms increases. This is discussed in more detail in the next section.

PROTECTIVE REFLEXES FROM MECHANORECEPTORS: DO THEY EXIST AND ARE THEY USEFUL IN MANIPULATION?

One working hypothesis of manual therapy is that short-latency protective reflexes or segmental reflexes can be used to infiltrate and influence the nervous system. For example, if a joint is overstretched, the Golgi tendon organs will inhibit the supposedly overactive antagonist muscles. In the light of current neurological

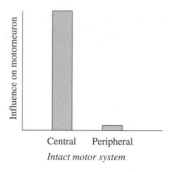

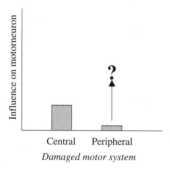

Figure 8.19   In the intact motor system, central influences are stronger than peripheral ones. The relationship may change following central damage of the motor system.

knowledge, it now seems that this proposed pathway is unrealistic.

Spindle afferents and the tendon reflex

The tendon reflex is not a part of the protective reflex system. As has been mentioned earlier, it is a physiological artefact that is unlikely to occur in normal reflex adjustments to sudden disturbances of movement. For example, when the foot collides with an obstacle during walking, the normal evasive reflex reaction is to flex the knee and hip to stay clear of the obstacle. If, as has been suggested, the tendon reflex were activated by the collision, it would mean that the sudden stretch of the quadriceps (brought on by the collision) would result in reflex extension of the knee. This would result in the foot jamming further into the obstacle. Others have reached the same conclusion with respect to the upper limbs. As with the lower limb, if the

movement of the arm is suddenly disturbed by an obstacle, it would be advantageous for the muscle to yield rather than become stiffer, which would be the situation if the reflex arc were strongly activated.[27]

Another widely held belief is that the tendon reflex plays a part in protecting muscles against excessive stretching. Against this notion stands the common finding that relaxed muscles can be stretched extensively without eliciting a reflex contraction. When, for example, the hamstring is passively stretched, there is no sudden reflex contraction of the muscle to protect it from damage. If that were the case, it would never be possible to elongate shortened muscles in treatment or exercise. Furthermore, if during high-velocity strain of a joint the stretched muscle were suddenly to contract, this would increase the tension on its series elastic component, resulting in greater strain and damage. Any reflex contraction brought on by stretching is probably a result of pain.

Normal adjustments to movement are much more complex than the tendon reflexes produced by manipulation. This implies that manual techniques such as high-velocity thrusts that produce a sudden stretch of the muscle–tendon unit are unlikely to influence motor processes.

Golgi tendon organs

It has been suggested that Golgi tendon organs act as sensors to protect the muscle from damage caused by excessive high-force contraction. There is a widely held belief that muscle stretching will activate the Golgi tendon organ to inhibit its own muscle. Such events never happen in real life. One can imagine what would happen were the Golgi afferents to inhibit the motorneurons to the arm during heavy lifting or, even worse, in a life-threatening situation such as hanging over a side of a cliff. This is supported by the fact that, during sports activities, one can tear a muscle during high-force contraction without a hint of a protective reflex. The Golgi tendon organ has only a mild influence over motor activities but cannot control central motor drives. The motivation for the evasive behaviour needed to protect the muscle is elicited by fatigue and pain.

Joint afferents

It has been proposed that techniques that stretch the joint will have an inhibitory influence on the muscles acting around the joint. This inhibitory mechanism is very unlikely to exist or be a viable method of reducing motor tone. To start with, the reflex inhibition brought about by joint afferents is very mild. Furthermore, the whole issue of protective reflexes arising from joint afferents has been put into question. It has been demonstrated that the reflex pathway of joint afferents is too slow to mediate protective reflexes in situations such as tripping during running and walking.[53,62] This is supported by the fact that a joint can be stretched during manipulation or exercise without any reflex activity of its relevant muscles unless the stretches involve pain. However, in this situation, the reflex response is muscular contraction rather than inhibition.

Can the tendon reflex be used in rehabilitation?

The proposed fallacy that proprioceptive feedback can be used to alter motor activity can be exemplified by a simple question: can stimulation of the quadriceps stretch reflex be used to rehabilitate knee extension during walking? Such rehabilitation would be highly unlikely for the following reasons:

1. The tendon reflex is a physiological artefact that does not occur during normal movement.
2. The tendon reflex is too weak to improve the force of contraction or muscle endurance.
3. The tendon reflex will fail to meet the patterns for normal/functional motor learning
4. Stimulating reflexes that are fragments of activity initiated from the periphery in a 'centripetal' direction cannot rehabilitate whole movement patterns that are initiated 'centrifugally', i.e. from the centre outwards.

DOES PERIPHERALLY MEDIATED RECIPROCAL INHIBITION HAVE A PLACE IN REHABILITATION?

When eliciting the stretch reflex in agonists, there is an observable drop in the antagonist EMG amplitude and contraction force. Various manual disciplines claim to be able to reduce abnormal motor tone by the activation of reciprocal inhibition. However, peripherally mediated inhibition has several limitations and may not be effective in influencing neural processes. These limitations are discussed below.

Duration of inhibition

Both the excitatory and the inhibitory response are of an extremely short duration. For example, in the interosseous muscles of the hand, stimulation of the stretch reflex will produce an excitatory response (combining the M1 and M2 latencies) with an overall duration of anywhere from 40 ms to 50 ms.[108] Inhibition of the antagonist may exhibit a similar duration.[82] At the end of this reflex, the activity in the motorneuron pool returns immediately to its prestimulation level. To tonically induce inhibition, the agonists have to be stimulated by either continuous agonist contraction or vibration. However, continuous vibration of the agonists sometimes produces only a transient reciprocal inhibition.[82]

Contraction force

The reduction in the contraction force of the antagonist muscles brought on by reciprocal inhibition is only 2–4%[82] of the agonist's contraction force; i.e. it is an extremely low-level reflex change of contraction force.[34] Reciprocal inhibition is therefore an extremely weak mechanism for reducing abnormal antagonist tone.

Latency of response

During arm movements the agonist muscles contract and the antagonists relax. Both excitation and inhibition must occur more or less simultaneously for coordination of the movement. If inhibition were mediated by the periphery (mechanoreceptors), the antagonist response would always lag behind the excitatory response. The lag in time of the response would result from a long sequence of neural events: the motor drive stimulating the intra- and extrafusal fibres of the agonist, followed by muscle contraction and stimulation of the spindle afferents; the signal from the afferents travelling back to the spinal cord and passing two or more interneurons, to finally, and with a considerable lag, inhibit the antagonist motorneuron pool. Indeed, when the tendon of flexor carpi radialis is vibrated or tapped, the reduced EMG activity from the antagonistic muscle occurs at a latency of 40 ms with a reduction in the force of contraction at a latency of 60 ms. This latency in the antagonists is some 40 ms after the onset of the M1 response in the agonist.[82] In real life, the motor drives to the agonist and antagonist motorneurons occur simultaneously and are probably regulated by central rather than peripheral mechanisms.[82]

Since the tendon reflex is considered to be a physiological artefact, this implies that reciprocal inhibition is also a physiological artefact; such reflexes may not be present during normal functional movement.

Co-contraction of agonists and antagonists

Agonist/antagonist inhibition is not present in all movements, many involving co-contraction of the agonist/antagonist muscle groups.[109] This means that treatment concentrating on patterns of reciprocal inhibition, by stimulation of receptors or even by central inhibition, will not transfer well to movement patterns that require co-contraction.

In manual techniques that utilize agonist/antagonist inhibition, the main contribution to inhibition of the antagonist muscles is central motor control, with possibly a faint inhibitory contribution from peripheral mechanisms.

In the treatment of spasticity, *central* inhibitory techniques are probably more efficient, functionally similar to movement and of longer duration than peripheral inhibition, as for example, in the use of neck rotation to inhibit muscle spasm in the upper extremity, or guiding the patient to relax a group of overactive muscles. These types of inhibitory technique are probably more important than reflexive peripheral techniques as they stimulate the whole motor system in functional patterns that resemble normal motor activity. These techniques are discussed in more detail in this section.

CONCLUSION: MANUAL TECHNIQUES CANNOT BE USED REFLEXIVELY TO CONTROL MOTOR ACTIVITY

Some of the reasons behind the above conclusion are summarized below (see also Fig. 8.20):

1. Afferents work in ensembles; no single group of receptors can be exclusively stimulated by manipulation.
2. The reflexogenic effect of proprioceptors is very mild in comparison with that of descending motor influences. Proprioceptors cannot control the gain of the motorneuron.
3. The reflex response (inhibition or excitation) is transient, existing only during manipulation.
4. Single episodes of manipulation, producing single reflex responses, are not sufficient to promote plastic adaptation in the motor system.

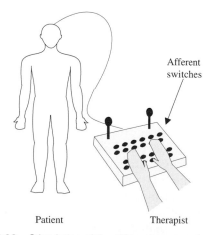

Patient   Therapist

Figure 8.20 Stimulation of the different groups of mechanoreceptor cannot act as a switch to control muscle activity. Muscle tone neurological origin cannot be switched on and off, or 'dimmed', by passive forms of manipulation.

5. There may be habituation of the reflex response to repeated stimulation, leading to a progressively decreasing reflex response.

6. The process is task dependent: any reflex response is heavily modulated by descending influences from higher centres, altering for different positions and movements. For example, the position of the head and arms can influence the excitability of the stretch reflex in the thigh. Rotation of the head to the right or left will increase or depress the reflex response.[110] The variations in reflex activity are probably as diverse as posture and are therefore infinite and unpredictable.

7. The peripherally induced reflex response (e.g. the tendon reflex) does not occur in normal motor activity. Many of these reflexes are experimentally produced physiological artefacts and will not transfer to normal functional movement, i.e. the reflex response has no functional motor meaning. It is not matched for correction of movement patterns, nor will it aid the learning of movement patterns.

8. In some situations, such as in central damage, repeated stimulation of abnormal reflexes may in time lead to augmentation of those reflexes (by neuroplasticity). This will be counterproductive to the rehabilitation of normal functional movement.

9. Most reflex-inducing treatments are carried out when the patient is relaxed. Any sensory feedback will be treated by the motor system as noise and will be discarded.

10. The motor system is not muscle or joint specific. During normal activity, even small movements of single joints will result in wholebody compensation occurring over many joints and muscle groups. Reflex activation or inhibition of one group of muscles cannot predict this complexity and enormity of movement.[111] One can only work with gross overall patterns.

11. Reflex-inducing techniques are only useful when there is central damage. In these circumstances, they can be used to break abnormal muscle activity so that movement that is functional and useful can be rehabilitated (see below). However, they cannot be used to rehabilitate normal functional movement.

In summary, controlling the motor system via the activation of peripheral mechanisms and segmental reflexes is equivalent to attempting to change the flow of a river by throwing a pebble into it. The next chapter proposes alternative models of how manipulation can be used to affect the motor system.

9

Motor learning, manual therapy and rehabilitation

In the previous chapter, the concept that the patient's nervous system can be controlled by peripheral events was challenged. An alternative model, is proposed here for the role of manipulation in influencing motor processes. In this model, the patient is actively and cognitively taking part in shaping the response with the aid of manual guidance. Rehabilitation provides the functional stimulus needed for regeneration (healing) and plasticity of the nervous system following injury. The key to change in function is motor learning and neuromuscular plasticity.

Much of the information in this section has been derived from concepts of and research into motor learning. However, neurophysiological mechanisms that underlie rehabilitation and motor learning are not entirely comparable. Motor learning relates largely to the acquisition of novel motor skills in healthy individuals. In rehabilitation, relearning a skill may not be novel, as the patient had experienced the motor event previous to the injury. However, the patient may not be capable of carrying out the movement. This may be due to some discontinuity within the motor system rather than to forgetfulness or damage to the memory centres. For example, a stroke patient who is unable to use the arm for writing has not forgotten how to write as a result of memory centre damage. The patient may be totally aware of the movement to be performed, but, because of the discontinuity of the system, is not able to carry out the movement. In much the same way, following damage to the knee joint, proprioception and balance on the damaged leg may be affected. In this condition, what has suddenly been lost is not the memory for balance but rather the proprioceptive feedback that contributes to it.

For much of the twentieth century, the models for neurorehabilitation derived from studies of the reflex activity in anaesthetized animal or animals with a partial motor system. This often has very little to do with rehabilitation or motor learning in humans. Although in the middle of the twentieth century, a vast research drive was undertaken in the area of psychology in motor learning, little of it has filtered into the different rehabilitation disciplines. More research is therefore needed to identify which principles of motor learning can contribute to neurorehabilitation.

PHASES OF MOTOR LEARNING

The different phases of motor learning are not distinct phases but rather a continuum and a progression of skill learning from a cognitive and high level of consciousness to a more subconscious automated activity.[112] The model for motor learning presented here is a synthesis of several models, in which motor learning is characterized by three phases:[113]

- cognitive phase
- associative phase
- autonomous phase.

Cognitive phase

This phase is marked by the high level of intellectual activity needed to understand the task that is being learned. For example, learning to drive a car will initially involve intense concentration to control the complex coordination of the limbs. In this stage, fragments of previous skills and abilities, some of which may be at an automatic level (Fig. 9.1),[112] are patched together to form the new skill.[113] Using the driving example, motor patterns used for sitting may be automatic, brought in from previous movement experiences, whereas limb movements may be novel patterns.

The cognitive stage also involves a higher degree of error in performance. Although the

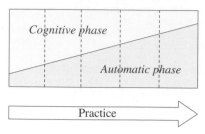

Figure 9.1 The progression of motor learning from the cognitive to the automatic phase. With practice, there is a shift in relationship of the two phases.

individual is aware of doing something wrong, he or she may not understand how the movement could be corrected and improved.[112] This is the reason for manual guidance at the cognitive stage, in which the therapist can give physical or verbal feedback to the patient on how to correct the movement. Guidance should progressively decrease as the movement pattern is becoming error free and more automatic.

Associative phase

This is an intermediate stage during which the newly acquired skill is executed and tested as a continuous whole pattern (whereas in the cognitive phase, it is still fragmented). This pattern is not fully without its faults and needs to be tried out, tested and readjusted.[113]

Autonomous phase

As the individual becomes more proficient in performing the skill, it becomes more automatic and less under conscious control. In this phase, the skill is stored as a motor programme and is more 'robust' to interference from other ongoing activities and environmental disturbances. Whereas in the cognitive stage subjects cannot perform two activities simultaneously, for example driving a car while talking, they may be able to do so in the autonomous phase.[114] Automatic activity may not be totally subconscious, and some elements of the movement may be on a cognitive level (Fig. 9.1).[112]

Learning phases can be observed in most rehabilitation processes. Initially, the patient's

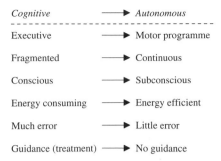

Figure 9.2 Some common features in the stages of motor learning.

ability to produce movement will be inaccurate and require intense concentration (Fig. 9.2). With time and repetition, the movement becomes more fluent, the patient being able to execute the movement automatically while, say, conversing with the therapist. Providing the patient is moving correctly, this should be encouraged as it may help to 'automate' the movement. For example, during their rehabilitation, stroke patients can be instructed to initiate free-arm swinging (imitating the rhythmic arm swings during walking). As the movement becomes more automatic, the patient can be encouraged to talk while swinging the arms.

Neurorehabilitation *must be initiated in the cognitive phase*; it cannot be initiated in the autonomous (automatic phase). This further implies that, without cognition and volition, a passive and reflexive treatment would have minimal or no effect on neurological processes (Fig. 9.3).

PLASTICITY IN THE MOTOR SYSTEM

Learning implies that the motor system is not fixed but has the capacity to store and adapt to new experiences. This ability of the motor system to undergo such changes is termed neuromuscular plasticity, indicating a simultaneous peripheral–muscular and central–neural adaptation. The understanding of the mechanisms that promote plasticity in the motor system is probably the most important element in any rehabilitation programme. Treatment that does not 'conform' to these mechanisms will be shortlasting and ineffective.

SPECIFICITY AND PLASTICITY

The view of the nervous system as a fixed functional and anatomical organization has been continuously challenged. The nervous system is now seen as capable of long-term readjustment in response to environmental demands. In order for an animal to be able to respond to the environment, it must be capable of two basic properties.[115] First, it must retain the stability of many functions in the face of the ever-changing environment. This is where specificity comes into play, where many functional activities of the nervous system are 'prewired' or 'hard-wired'.[115] This kind of organization offers a background stability and certainty to many of our daily activities. However, an organism endowed with only specificity will not be able to adapt to new

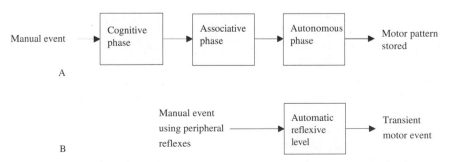

Figure 9.3 (A) A manual event that follows normal motor learning patterns will be stored as part of the motor repertoire. (B) Reflexive-type manipulation will have only a transient effect.

situations that arise in its changing environment. To be able to adapt to new experiences, the animal must also have the potential for plasticity,[115] which is mediated within the CNS by various mechanisms (Fig. 9.4):[2,115,116]

- changes in the neuronal cell surface and its filaments
- growth of new synaptic connections
- sprouting of cell dendrites and axons
- changes in neurotransmitter release at synapses
- following injury, the regeneration of neural tissue.

STUDIES OF PLASTICITY IN THE MOTOR SYSTEM

Motor learning is marked by the capacity of the motor system to undergo adaptive and plastic changes. Motor adaptation is a perpetual process carried out throughout life and is not limited to young animals.

Plasticity in the motor system is well documented. Studies have demonstrated that the cortical representation of the sensorimotor cortex can change in the intact nervous system of an adult animal. For example, tapping the index and middle finger of a monkey daily for several months changes the cortical representation of the hand. The region of the cortex area representing the hand will increase, distorting the map in favour of the tapped fingers.[116] Such changes can be also observed in humans. In blind Braille readers, there is an expansion of the sensorimotor cortical representation of the reading finger.[117]

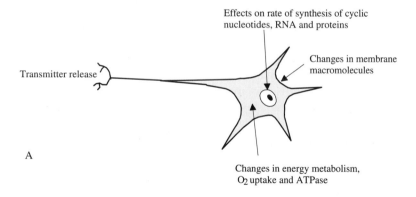

Figure 9.4 Structural and physiological changes underlying neuroplasticity. (A) Key stages of short-term memory (about a few seconds post-stimulation). (B) Key stages of long-term memory (about 3–20 minutes post-stimulation).

Sensorimotor plasticity can also be demonstrated following injury. In normal circumstances, because the palm of the hand is used more than the dorsum, the median nerve has a greater cortical representation. When the median nerve is cut, the cortical map of the hand changes in size in favour of the intact radial nerve. If the median nerve is allowed to regenerate, it will recapture some of its lost cortical territory. Similarly, amputees or patients with spinal cord injuries show a lower threshold of excitation of muscles proximal to the lesion.[118] Changes in excitability are attributed to enlarged sensorimotor representation of the unaffected proximal muscle, whilst the sensorimotor representation of the unused muscles below the lesion has reduced in size.

Plastic changes have been shown to take place even in the most simple pathways such as the monosynaptic stretch reflex. Monkeys can be trained by the offer of a reward to depress or elevate the EMG amplitude of the stretch reflex.[119–121] Plastic changes of the stretch reflex will occur after a few weeks to a few months and will persist for long periods of time, even after the removal of supraspinal influences.[121] This implies that the spinal cord has the capacity to store movement patterns. (Although the stretch reflex was elicited by the stimulation of afferents, the adaptive drive was mediated by the higher centres.) In humans, similar plastic changes of the stretch reflex can be demonstrated, the main difference being the time it takes to induce them. Whereas in a monkey it may take a few weeks, in humans such changes are observable after only nine sessions.[122] The reason for this difference may lie in the potent influence that cognition has in humans in accelerating the learning process.

Motor learning has also been shown in animals that have only their spinal cord intact.[123] These animals are taught to either stand or walk using their hindlimbs. The animals that were taught to stand could use their hindlimbs for that purpose but were unable to produce locomotor movement patterns. Conversely, animals who were taught to walk could produce the muscular activity necessary for walking but were poor at standing. These two conditions could be reversed by training each group in the other motor task; i.e. the walking group could be trained to stand, and vice versa. Once the activity was changed, the animal was unable to perform the previous motor task. These experiments highlight two important factors:

1. that plasticity is not centre specific but tends to occur at different levels within the motor system[124]
2. that the motor system is highly specific when learning motor tasks.

MEMORY STORES

Sensory experiences may or may not be stored in the CNS depending on various conditions. In this respect, one can speak of three memory potentials (Fig. 9.5):[3,112]

- short-term sensory store
- short-term memory
- long-term memory.

These memory potentials are not discrete systems but part of a memory continuum in which a sensory experience may proceed to be stored in the long term or made redundant at a very early stage of the experience.

Short-term sensory store

The sensory store is the sustaining of sensory information within the system immediately after stimulation. This information is maintained for a very short period, lasting between 250 ms and 2 seconds, before it is replaced by the next stream of sensory information.[3,113] The capacity and duration are heavily affected by the complexity of the information and the succeeding patterns of information.

Within the vast input of sensory information, the nervous system can select different streams of information depending on the importance and relevance of the information to the task. The ability of the motor system to choose the most relevant stream of sensory information is called *selective attention*,[112] and will also affect the length of retention of the sensory event.[125]

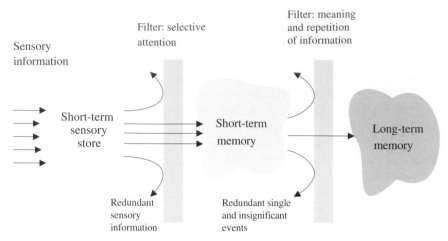

Figure 9.5 A functional model of memory stores.

Short-term memory

Once a stimulus has been processed, it will retain information only as long as attention is drawn to it by reciting or repetition of movement. Memory of a motor response follows a similar pattern to that of verbal memory, a memory trace of a motor response decaying rapidly in a matter of seconds but becoming more stable with reinforcement of the same activity.[126] Without repetition verbal information has been shown to be lost within 30 seconds.[113] In motor learning, it was demonstrated that, with one rehearsal, the degree of error after 120 seconds almost doubled. Fifteen rehearsals reduced the degree of error at this time interval by half. This is very important to the rehabilitation process: *a single motor event or manipulation will be lost very rapidly if not repeated over and over again*.[3] Table 9.1 highlights the importance of repetition in neurorehabilitation. Because treatment is not sufficient to fulfil the repetition 'quota,' it will need to be complemented by exercise and functional movement outside treatment sessions.

Long-term memory

The encoding of the information from the short- to the long-term memory requires repetition or to have a meaningful content (Table 9.1). Once the pattern has been stored in the long-term memory, it will not be lost in the absence of rehearsal. Indeed, this can be observed in repetitive motor acts such as swimming, cycling or playing a musical instrument.[3] One can perform many of these skills after many years without much practice.

Meaning and emotion can change the need for repetition. For example, being punched does not require much repetition for the event to be memorized (as I can unfortunately confirm), whereas accidentally knocking one's head is rarely remembered, even in fairly severe physical trauma. Experiences with strong emotional significance are almost always transferred from the short- to the long-term memory.[3]

Table 9.1 Estimated number of repetitions needed to achieve skilled performance

Activity	Repetition for skilled performance
Cigar-making	3 million cigars
Hand knitting	1.5 million stitches
Rug-making	1.4 million knots
Violin playing	2.5 million notes
Walking, up to 6 years	3 million steps
Marching	0.8 million steps
Pearl-handling	1.5–3 million
Football passing	1.4 million passes
Basketball playing	1 million baskets
Gymnast performing	8 years daily practice

After Kottke et al 1978 with permission from W. B. Saunders.[127]

THE PLASTIC/ADAPTIVE CODE IN REHABILITATION OF THE MOTOR SYSTEM

In reality, we retain only a small fraction of what we receive from our senses. Not all experiences are meaningful or important to our survival and function, and will therefore have little or no influence on neural adaptation. Some sensorimotor experiences will be stored whilst others will become redundant and lost. Understanding why some experiences are retained as learning and how others are discarded is very important for rehabilitation.

The elements in a movement pattern that promote plasticity can be likened to a code: experiences that possess a higher content of adaptive code elements have a greater potential for promoting long-term plastic changes. Experiences with a low adaptive code content will fail to promote any significant adaptation. The adaptive code, therefore, is the code that encourages long-term retention and learning of physical and mental activity. Failure to imitate this form of stimulus will result in an ineffective, short-lived response to treatment.

Plasticity associated with motor development in learning and following neural damage is driven by comparable neuronal processes.[120] The difference may be only in the 'scale, address and connectivity'.[129] This is very convenient to the therapist as treatment will be very similar almost regardless of the type of neurological dysfunction, whether it is rehabilitation of a peripheral joint after injury, development of postural awareness or treating patients with central damage after a stroke. If these dysfunctions require similar treatments, there must be similar basic elements underlying these treatments. Some of these variables are listed below (Fig. 9.6):

- *Cognitive/volitional rather than reflexive*: Changes in the motor system can only be achieved by following the sequence of motor learning.
- *Repetition of manual event*: Repetition should be used during the same session and over consecutive sessions. Whenever possible, the patient

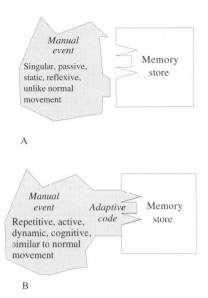

Figure 9.6   Schematic representation of the adaptive code. (A) Manual events low on adaptive code elements are unlikely to be stored as a memory trace. (B) Manual events containing adaptive code elements have a greater potential to promote long-term plastic changes.

should be encouraged to repeat the activity during daily activity or complement it by exercise.

- *Transfer*: Treatment should mimic intended skill or lost motor ability to facilitate motor transfer (see below).
- *Active rather than passive technique*: Use active rather than passive techniques (if possible) to engage the complete motor system. This is discussed in more detail in the section below on manual guidance.
- *Dynamic rather than static technique*: Dynamic techniques closely resemble functional movement and motor transfer may therefore be greater than in static techniques.
- *Communication*: Use verbal and visual communication in treatment. For example, encourage the patient to visualize the movement or verbally guide the patient on how to relax before, during or following movement. Explain the goal and purpose of the movement.

PRINCIPLES IN MOTOR LEARNING

TRANSFER OF TRAINING

Any activity that has been learned during the treatment session ultimately has to support the patient in a variety of daily activities.[130] For example, if the use of the arm is being rehabilitated, the motor learning achieved during the treatment session should hopefully transfer into activities such as eating.

Transfer has been defined as 'the effect that practice of one task has upon the learning or performance of a second task'.[13] Motor transfer relies on various elements, one of which is the sameness of the motor task:[131] the closer the training is to the intended task, the greater the transfer will be.[132] For example, being able to type does not necessarily transfer to playing a piano. To play the piano, one needs repeatedly to practise playing a piano.

For motor guidance to be effective, the principles of transfer should be incorporated into the treatment programme. Rehabilitation should include movements that are closely related to the intended task. The closer the movement is to the intended task, the greater the transfer will be. These movement patterns should also be combined with movements that are 'around' or a variation of the task. This may initially seem to produce confusion and add little to the transfer, but, in time, this form of learning will produce flexibility in the variety of performance.[131] Subjects who are given the full range of possible movement patterns have less error in producing the task than do subjects who are shown the correct path.[131] Different variables, such as speed of movement, force and combination of movements, can be used to enlarge the motor repertoire. For example, if arm abduction is being rehabilitated, the treatment programme could involve arm abduction movements (a similar task) with, say, abduction in external and internal rotation or varying degrees of flexion and extension (a variation of the task). Tasks and movement patterns that are too similar and lack variety may induce boredom in both patient and therapist, thus reducing attention during treatment and impeding learning.

MOTOR ABILITIES AND SKILLS

The transfer principle raises an important question about the rehabilitation programme. Should rehabilitation imitate daily tasks or should it be broken down into elements that make up whole movement? This question brings rehabilitation into the ability–skill distinction.

Abilities are the motor traits of the individual that underlie any physical activity.[133,134] An acrobat walking on a tightrope depends on the basic ability of balance and coordination. A musician may rely on the abilities of manual dexterity, coordination and speed to play a musical instrument. In the martial arts, an individual who shows good speed will be expected to perform better than an individual with low speed ability.[13] Motor abilities are a mixture of genetic traits and the products of learning that develop during childhood and adolescence.[133,134] Once the motor system has matured in adult life, these abilities become more permanent and are more difficult to change. However, it has been argued that abilities remain flexible through life and can be affected by practice.[113,135] High-level ability in different areas will contribute to proficiency in the performance of different skills.[136–138] Some of the abilities that underlie motor activity are summarized in Table 9.2.[133,134]

Skill refers to how well a person can perform a given task. Proficiency in performing any skill is dependent partly on the individual's motor abilities and partly on rehearsal. Many new learned skills are made up of fragments of previous skills synthesized together to form a new movement pattern. This means that, after the first few years of motor development, only a few skills are totally new.

How abilities underlie motor learning can be seen when an individual learns a novel skill. For example, when learning to play a piano or type, the whole skill of playing is broken into ability components. Initially, only a few keys will be played in a sequence. This represents a learning drive towards improving the abilities of fine

Table 9.2   The different ability traits and muscle recruitment patterns involved in physical activity. Some of these techniques are described further in Fig. 9.7

Abilities underlying physical skill	Description	Ability-enhancing manual techniques
Multilimb coordination	Ability to coordinate a number of limbs simultaneously	Active–dynamic technique involving whole body movement patterns such as used in PNF
Response orientation	Directional discrimination and orientation of movement pattern	Patient follows movement patterns initiated by therapist. Increase proprioceptive acuity by instructing the patient to close the eyes
Reaction time	Time lapse between stimulus and patient's response	Patient is instructed to react as fast as possible to a change in the therapist's guiding hand or a verbal cue; e.g. therapist guides patient's arm into flexion and, when stimulus is given, patient has to quickly change direction of movement
Speed of movement	Speed of gross limb movement when accuracy not required	Active dynamic techniques with rapid rate of movement, e.g. rapid extension or flexion of knee to set position such as the therapist's hand. Change position of hand to produce small to large arcs of movement or direction of movement
Rate control	Ability to make continuous motor adjustments relative to changes in speed and direction of an object	Active dynamic techniques with continuous varying force speed and direction imposed by therapist
Control precision	Ability to hold steady position coupled with fine movements of limbs and hands Important in operation of equipment where rapid, precise use of control is required	Patient stands on good leg and, with injured leg, draws numbers 1 to 10. Or, patient lying follows movement imposed by therapist using injured leg
Balance	Ability to use limbs or whole body in standing and movement	Patient stands on injured leg. Therapist supports patient but gently moves patient off balance. Alter knee flexion angle, ask patient to stand on toes or heel and balance
Introspect/kinesthesis and relax	Ability to 'see' proprioceptively and refine motor activity	1. Gentle passive movement of limb (e.g. shoulder and arm), palpating for tension in muscles and providing patient with verbal feedback on the level of relaxation in muscles 2. Patient fully contracts the tense muscle and then relaxes. Patient is instructed to concentrate on state of tension during contraction phase and on muscle relaxation following it

Rehabilitation programme can also include techniques that enhance central control together with local physical state of muscle:

Static strength	Isometric strength of muscle	Active–static technique, different level of force applied at different angles, e.g. 50°, 90° knee flexion or any other angle. Add internal and external knee rotation or hip rotation
Dynamic strength	Muscle strength during movement	As above in static strength, but resistance to movement is through a dynamic range
Explosive strength	Ability to exert maximum energy in one explosive act such as a short sprint	Important in sports rehabilitation. Remedial exercise such as throwing an object as far or as high as possible
Dynamic flexibility	Extent of flexibility during active movement, e.g. passive rotation of cervical spine is greater than active	E.g. holding patient's head, instruct patient to fully rotate to end-range, adding some resistance throughout range. Repeat at different velocities

Table 9.2 *(contd)*

Abilities underlying physical skill	Description	Ability-enhancing manual techniques
To the above motor abilities, other physiological mechanisms of muscle group recruitment can be added to the rehabilitation programme:		
Antagonist co-activation	Co-contraction of two antagonistic group of muscle, e.g. hamstring and quadriceps	Instruct patient to stiffen knee and resist rapid application of flexion and extension cycles
Reciprocal activation	Activation of one muscle group while its antagonist pair is relaxed	Instruct patient to extend then flex leg against resistance. At end of each movement, before limb is about to move in opposite direction, instruct patient to fully relax the prime mover. Vary level of resistance and speed of change between muscle groups. Also change joint angles

PNF, Proprioceptive neuromuscular facilitation.

control and precision. A gradual increase in the speed of playing represents an improvement in speed ability.

MOTOR ABILITIES IN REHABILITATION

Rehabilitation is ultimately directed towards helping the patient to regain normal motor activity in work and leisure. The rehabilitation programme has to acknowledge the activity to which the patient will return. Rehabilitation of a sports injury will concentrate on specific groups of motor ability underlying the particular activity, for example the ability to use explosive force for tennis serves. This will be different from the rehabilitation of an office worker suffering from a repetitive strain injury.

Improving abilities during the treatment period may reduce the need to rehabilitate all of the patient's daily skills. A stroke patient will not be guided through all the possible daily tasks but, instead, though certain underlying abilities that will help to improve a variety of skills. Treatment may encompass such abilities as coordination, static force, dynamic force and control precision. This does not exclude the rehabilitation of specific skills that contain elements of the lost abilities. Many of these abilities can be reinforced by encouraging the patient to perform daily tasks that depend on these abilities.

The motor programme and its neuromuscular connection will adapt to the activity in which it was trained (see the sections on neuroplasticity and transfer above).[139] For example, if motor learning involves static force ability, the person may improve that area but not necessarily speed or coordination. If these are to develop, they must be included in the rehabilitation programme. If the aim of treatment is to rehabilitate balance, balance-enhancing techniques must be used; muscle force enhancement techniques alone will not be sufficient. This point is very important, as musculoskeletal rehabilitation often focuses on force rehabilitation regardless of the activity to which the patient is returning. This principle is highlighted by the following example. Teaching a child to write involves endless repetitions to improve such abilities as speed, finger precision, coordination and force in the form of endurance. Training in force ability in this situation would be inconceivable: it is unthinkable for the child to perform warming-up finger force exercises using weights. In much the same way, a person who has suffered a stroke may be unable to write because of loss of strength, fine control and coordination. Treatment that focuses on strength exercise alone will be of only limited benefit. Unless coordination and precision are redeveloped, the person will be unable to write, no matter how strong his or her muscles are.

Motor abilities in the treatment of musculoskeletal injury

An indication of the importance of abilities following musculoskeletal injury has been assessed in the rehabilitation of subjects with anterior cruciate ligament damage in the knee.[140] One group received the commonly prescribed treatment of active–static techniques, whilst the other carried out a programme designed to enhance proprioception. This programme included active–dynamic exercise and the use of repetition, speed, balance, coordination and movement patterns. Although in both programmes there was an improvement in function, this improvement was significantly greater in the proprioceptive group. Similarly, functional instability of the ankle was shown to improve with treatment that focused on improving functional movement, balance and coordination ability. The improvement in the group working on abilities was significantly greater than that of the group receiving conventional treatment.[141]

INTROSPECTIVE/AWARENESS AND RELAXATION ABILITIES

Added to the list of abilities that can be improved during treatment are introspection/awareness and relaxation ability, which are important for postural and movement awareness and motor relaxation. Some patients seem unable to introspect and 'feel their body', and may find it difficult to relax fully.[142] This inability may impede the rate of improvement.

PHYSIOLOGICAL ABILITIES: RECIPROCAL ACTIVATION AND ANTAGONIST CO-ACTIVATION

Reciprocal activation and antagonist co-activation are patterns of motor recruitment in muscles. Although these are strictly not motor abilities, abnormal motor activity may result from changes in the patterns of motor recruitment.

Antagonist co-activation is a motor pattern that serves partly to increase the stiffness and stability of joints during static posture and movement.[62,143,144] In co-activation, antagonistic muscle groups (e.g. the hamstrings and quadriceps) contract simultaneously. Reciprocal activation, in which the agonist group is contracting while the antagonist group is passively elongated serves to produce movement. During various motor activities, these patterns of contraction take place either separately or jointly. For example, during intricate physical activity such as using a pair of scissors, co-activation stabilizes the whole limb and hand while reciprocal activation produces the cutting movement.[109] These two forms of activation can be demonstrated during slow and fast joint movements. While sitting, if one slowly extends one's knee, reciprocal activation of the quadriceps and passive elongation of hamstrings can be felt. Co-activation can be felt when standing with the knees slightly flexed, in which position, both the hamstrings and quadriceps muscles will be working simultaneously.

It has been demonstrated that both forms of activation have separate motor control centres.[20,109] It has been suggested that the rigidity seen in patients with central motor damage may be attributed to malfunction of these centres.[109] The excessive muscle activity seen in these patients may possibly be related to increased co-activation. In failure of voluntary activation following joint damage, the inhibition and wasting of one group of muscles may alter the normal relationship between reciprocal and co-activation.

Patients can be guided on how to use the two modes of muscle recruitment (Fig. 9.7). For example, co-activation can be achieved by instructing the patient to stiffen the joint whilst the practitioner attempts to move the joint rapidly into cycles of extension and flexion. Other methods are to instruct the patient to oscillate the joint rapidly within a narrow range, and asking the patient to produce a full voluntary isotonic contraction. Reciprocal activation can be produced during different movements by instructing the patient to relax antagonistic muscle groups. It has also been demonstrated (although not in all patterns of movement) that co-activation virtually disappears when subjects

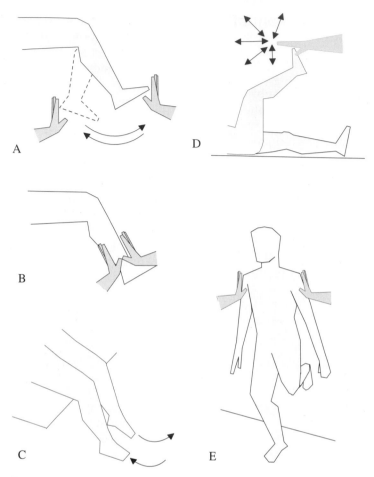

Figure 9.7 Manual guidance of some motor abilities. (A) Instruct the patient to oscillate the leg between your hands. Vary the speed of oscillation, changing the position and distance between your hands. (B) Hold the patient's leg firmly, instructing the patient to flex and extend the knee. Vary the force of contraction and the speed, and change the angle of the knee. (C) Alternate leg swings: vary the amplitude and speed. (D) Instruct the patient to follow your hand movement with the limb. Start with the patient's eyes open and then instruct the patient to close them. Vary the direction, speed and resistance to movement. (E) Stand behind the patient, providing support and instructing the patient to stand on one leg. Randomly move the patient off balance.

are instructed to relax at the initiation of movement.[145] Movement that is high in co-activation may shift towards reciprocal activation with practice.[146] This may be important for reducing mechanical stress and energy expenditure during movement.

ENERGY CONSERVATION IN MOVEMENT

Finer control and coordination in movement reduces the expenditure of energy and mechanical stresses on the musculoskeletal system.[147]

Refinement of movement increases the potential for a better recovery as well as reducing the eventuality for future damage to the system. Excessive coactivation may lead to an early onset of muscle fatigue, as the antagonistic muscles are acting against each other.

The efficiency of movement is related to patterns of inhibition and excitation during movement. Bobath has stated that 'each motor engram (program) is a pathway of excitation surrounded by a wall of inhibition'.[127] Indeed, the largest proportion of descending pathways are inhibitory.[53] Practice of a specific motor skill results in the excitation of the desired neuronal pathways with the inhibition of pathways that do not contribute to the movement.[127] However, in the early stages of learning, the inhibitory patterns may not be well developed, and 'nonproductive' muscle activity may lead to error and excessive energy consumption during movement. Such inhibition and excitation can be observed in the patterns of muscle recruitment during the early stages of motor learning (Fig. 9.8). At this stage, the new movement pattern is executed with excessive co-activation. With practice, muscle recruitment tends to be modified towards reciprocal activation, which is more fluent and energy efficient (demonstrating less overall muscle activity).[109,146,148] The change in the mode of recruitment is probably associated with improved inhibition of the antagonist muscles. This relationship between the refinement of movement and the expenditure of energy can be seen during many motor learning processes. For example, when learning to drive, one may during the first few lessons experience muscle fatigue and pain in the leg muscles. With practice, the movement of the feet on the pedals becomes more refined and effortless. If the motor system were unable to adapt and increase the efficiency of motor output, such high-energy activity would eventually lead to musculoskeletal failure.

GUIDED MOTOR IMAGERY

Guided motor imagery refers to the situation of a person imagining using the motor system but not producing any movement. Guided motor imagery can be used in two principle ways:

- facilitating motor learning
- motor relaxation.

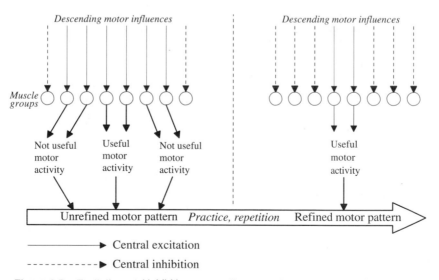

Figure 9.8 Excitation and inhibition as contributors to the conservation of energy in the motor system.

Facilitating motor learning

In much the same way that we mentally recite a numerical or verbal cue, physical action can also be improved by thinking about the movement.[131] This encourages the formation of internal connections within the motor system as well as preparing the motor programme for the ensuing activity.

When subjects are asked to visualize a motor activity such as hitting a nail with a hammer twice, but without carrying out the movement, the arm EMG trace will show two separate bursts of activity.[149] Similar efferent activity has been shown also to occur during simulation of other mental activities, such as climbing a rope or rowing. Although these EMG patterns are somewhat different from those of normal activity, they do suggest that a large portion of the motor system is engaged during the mental process.[3] A similar process takes place when we mentally recite words: the vocal muscles are minutely activated although no sound is produced.[149]

Physical activities that have been shown to improve by mental practice include bowling, piano playing and ball throwing. It has also been reported that mental practice can improve muscular endurance.[150] The effect of mental practice on motor performance was demonstrated in a study in which one group of subjects was given a novel motor task whilst another group rehearsed the task mentally, i.e. they only thought about the movement. The mental practice group was shown to be as effective as the physical practice group in the performance of the task after 10 days (Fig. 9.9).[151] More recently, it has been demonstrated that muscle strength can also be improved by mental practice.[152] The increase in force for the practice group was 30%, and for the mental practice group, 20%. The mechanisms that lie behind this force increase are related to the effect that mental practice has on the motor programme. During the initial period of muscle training, the gains achieved in force production are due not to muscle hypertrophy but to the more effective recruitment of the motorneurons supplying the

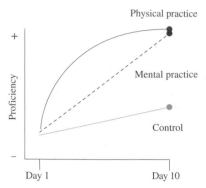

Figure 9.9   Proficiency on a tracking task. (After Rawings et al 1972.[151])

muscle (only after a few weeks of continuous practice will there be changes in the muscle tissue itself).

Guided motor imagery can be used in manual therapy, especially in situations where passive movement is being used (although this does not exclude the use of visualization in active techniques). Passive techniques alone may fail to engage the whole motor system (see below). However, encouraging patients to think about the movement during passive techniques may facilitate motor learning. The combination of passive movement and visualization may engage larger sections of the motor system, i.e. sensory feedback and the executive and effector levels (see Fig. 9.12).

Motor relaxation

Guided motor imagery can also be used to subdue the activity of the motor system, thus promoting general muscle relaxation. Motor relaxation techniques can be used before the initiation of movement, during or following the movement, in order to create movement that is less physically stressful and more energy efficient.

Motor relaxation can also be used in the rehabilitation of patients with central nervous system damage. It has been shown that patients suffering from spasticity can completely relax their overactive muscles (although this relaxation is only transient).[142] Relaxation can be used in these situations to break the spastic neuromuscular activity that impedes normal movement patterns. In this situation, an important connection is made between higher and spinal centres, although it may be an inhibitory one (see below).

Motor relaxation is also a motor learning process and is therefore governed by many of the principles of motor learning. It must start with a cognitive phase, often characterized by excessive mental effort and awareness of the errors being made in relaxation. With time and practice, this should lead to a phase in which relaxation is more automatic, rapid and requires less mental effort. Repetition of the relaxation within the same and subsequent sessions is very important to encourage long-term memory and automatization of the relaxation process. This must be combined with continuous and immediate feedback by the therapist, which provides the patient with feedback other than their own (patients are often not aware of tensing their muscles). For example, when guiding a patient to relax the neck muscle, the therapist's hands are used to continuously palpate and 'scan' the different muscle groups looking for changes in motor activity. Initially, the patient may find it difficult to maintain a relaxed state, tending to alternate between tension and relaxation. This changing state of the muscles is picked up by the palpating hand and is verbally conveyed to the patient. The principle of transfer is also important in motor relaxation. The ability to relax during the treatment session should be transferred to daily activities.[147]

There are numerous techniques for motor relaxation. For example, the patient may be instructed to introspect and relax different groups of muscles while the therapist is palpating the muscle and providing verbal feedback on the state of tension. Another common method is the contract–relax technique. The patient is instructed to contract against resistance while being given verbal instructions to feel the tension in the contracting muscle. He or she is then instructed to relax and is verbally instructed to compare the current state of relaxation with the previous state of contraction.

ENHANCING PROPRIOCEPTION

Within the sensory part of the motor system different sensory modalities can be enhanced in relationship to others, for example proprioception in proportion to other feedback elements such as vision. Conditions that may benefit from proprioception enhancement are discussed in Chapter 10. Proprioception can be enhanced by either:

- increasing the afferent volley by stimulation of the various mechanoreceptors
- reducing visual feedback.

Enhancing proprioception by afferent stimulation

Various groups of mechanoreceptors can be maximally stimulated to increase proprioception from different musculoskeletal structures. Skin mechanoreceptors can be maximally stimulated by dynamic events on the skin, for example massage, rubbing and vibration. Maximal stimulation of joint receptors can be achieved by articulation techniques such as cyclical rhythmical joint movement or oscillation. The awareness of a group of muscles can be achieved by instructing the patient cyclically to contract and relax the muscle. Alternatively, the patient can be instructed to contract isometrically while the therapist disturbs the held position by, for example, oscillating the joint. Generally speaking, active–dynamic techniques produce the largest proprioceptive inflow; second to these come passive–dynamic techniques.

Enhancing proprioception by reducing visual feedback

Proprioception can also be enhanced by reducing visual feedback during movement. In the normal process of motor learning, vision has a dominant influence over proprioception, which lessens as the task is learned and becomes automated. However, if vision is reduced early in the learning process, it increases the reliance of the subject on proprioception for correcting and learning the movement. When subjects are assessed for balance ability on a beam, those blindfolded relied heavily on proprioception, their performance being significantly better than subjects with complete or partial vision.[153] Reduced visual feedback has also been shown to be useful in remedial exercises following musculoskeletal injury.[140] In one such study of anterior cruciate ligament damage, many of the remedial exercises were performed with closed eyes to enhance proprioception from the damaged area. Enhancing proprioception with the aid of reduced visual feedback is often used in body/movement awareness disciplines such as yoga, the Feldenkreise method and Tai-Chi.

MANUAL GUIDANCE

The underlying concept in manual therapy that the motor system can be controlled by peripheral receptors cannot be sustained under current understanding of the motor system, as discussed above. The term 'guidance' rather than 'control' is more appropriate in describing the role of manipulation in rehabilitating the motor system. 'Guidance' is a term used in training and teaching, subjects being provided with knowledge of their results to enable them to modify their actions.[131] This helps to reduce error during the training period and facilitates the learning process. There are many forms of guidance, one of which is physical guidance. Manual neuro-rehabilitation can be viewed as a form of guidance, for example on helping a patient to regain the use of arm movements following musculoskeletal injury or stroke.

Much of the information in this section is derived from research into motor learning involving healthy subjects with an intact nervous system. It is assumed that many of the processes that underlie motor learning in healthy individuals can be inferred to those with different neuromuscular conditions.

ASSISTIVE AND RESISTIVE TECHNIQUES

Manual guidance can take two forms (Fig. 9.10):

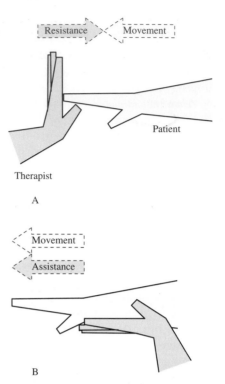

Figure 9.10 Resistive (A) and assistive (B) forms of guidance.

- *In resistive guidance*, the therapist resists the movement. This can be in a dynamic or a static pattern.
- *In assistive guidance*, movement is initiated by the patient and is aided by the therapist. Assistive guidance can be either passive, in which the movement is initiated and carried out by the therapist, or active, in which the patient is voluntarily moving with the aid of the therapist.

In general, guidance is useful during the remedial stage, but once the patient returns to normality, guidance should be reduced or totally removed and the patient should be encouraged to take over the rehabilitation process,[3] as prolonged guidance may cause over-reliance in the patient. This will, in the long term, have a detrimental effect on motor rehabilitation.[154,155]

THE INFLUENCE OF TECHNIQUE MODE ON MOTOR LEARNING

Particular techniques are more effective at influencing the motor system, so the choice of technique mode during guidance is very important. The neurophysiological response to the different modes of technique can be explored from several aspects:

- *afferent recruitment*: the number of receptors recruited and the change in their firing rate
- *proprioceptive acuity*: how well can subjects judge the position and movement of their limbs?
- *learning and transfer*: do the different modes and patterns of technique provide the necessary stimulus for motor learning? Can movement learned during guidance be used in daily activity?

PASSIVE AND ACTIVE TECHNIQUE

Passive and active techniques are regularly used in manual therapy for a wide range of clinical conditions. Surprisingly little research has been carried out to assess the differences between these two groups of techniques, although their potential difference may be very important to rehabilitation. On the whole, active techniques are probably more important than passive ones in neuromuscular rehabilitation. The differences are discussed below.

Afferent recruitment

The effect of different modes of technique on the afferent volley has been explored in Chapter 8. During active techniques, there is generally a greater afferent barrage than in passive techniques. This difference in recruitment is related to the activity of the muscle–tendon afferents during the two types of movement. In passive movement, the Golgi afferents are silent and the spindle primaries are firing at a low rate. In active movement, there is increased temporal and spatial activity as the Golgi tendon organs

and muscle spindles become more active. This has been demonstrated in a study in which proprioceptive acuity was compared in two intensities of actively resisted leg positioning; the higher intensity resulted in higher proprioceptive acuity.[74]

Proprioceptive acuity

It has been shown that movement detection by subjects is markedly better in active than in passive movement (Fig. 9.11).[75] When a subject's finger is moved passively, the ability to distinguish finger position is reduced compared with when the subject is instructed to stiffen the finger slightly during the movement.[72,156] It has been demonstrated in animals that the activity in the sensory cortex tends to increase and is more extensive during active than passive movement.[22] More extensive cortical activity may explain the increase in acuity associated with active movement.

It has also been proposed that the superiority of position sense in active motion is related to

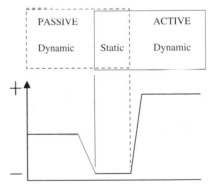

Proprioceptive awareness

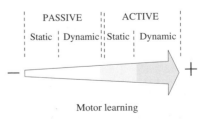

Motor learning

Figure 9.11 Different forms of manual guidance: their contribution to proprioception and motor learning.

the efferent flow and the 'sense of effort' that is internally derived within the CNS. This is an internal feedback mechanism occurring within the executive, effector and efferent copies and the comparator centre.[75] In active movement, therefore, feedback is derived from both proprioception and the internal feedback described above, which does not exist in passive motion. Passive movement will largely stimulate the feedback portion of the motor system and to some extent that of the executive level; i.e. it will fail to engage the total motor system. In comparison active techniques will engage all levels of the motor system (Fig. 9.12).

Learning and transfer

During active movement, the whole of the motor system is engaged, whereas during passive movement, there is no efferent activity or muscle recruitment.[157] It is therefore highly unlikely that passive movement can be encoded as a full motor pattern.

When vision is distorted by special lenses, the ability of the subject to learn to correct arm movement is greatly enhanced by active rather than passive arm movement.[36] This group of researchers have concluded that an active form of movement is a prerequisite for motor learning:

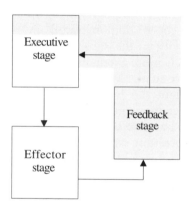

Passive technique

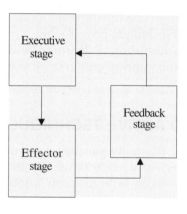

Active technique

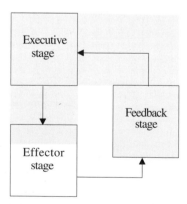

Passive with visualization of movement

Figure 9.12   The extent of involvement of the motor system in passive and active techniques and in passive technique with movement visualization.

'active movement yields highly significant adaptive effects whereas passive movement yields either significantly less adaptation or none at all'.[36] Matthews[16] has pointed out that, during normal daily activity, passive movement rarely occurs. (Since reading this comment, I have been trying to find passive movement in daily activity, without success.) It can be inferred from this simple observation that the motor system is well adapted to learn active rather than passive movement. Motor learning requires ongoing adjustments of motor activity in relation to the sensory input. Passive movement is not matched at the comparator level to any ongoing motor activity and would therefore not contribute to correction of movement or motor learning (Fig. 9.12).

The difference between active and passive movements can also be observed in human cognitive processes.[158] In maze training, one group received training that restricted their movements to the correct path, so that no choice was made. Another group was given choice while moving through the maze. Although both forms of guidance were active, the performance of the 'choice' group was greatly superior to that of the 'no-choice' group. Similarly, one may find that when driven to a new address, it is difficult to remember the route on recall. The rate of learning the route is facilitated when one is driving the car while finding the way using a map. A friend told me how for 3 years she was a passenger, driven by a friend to college. When she finally got her own car, she could not remember the route until she had actively driven it herself.

Manual implications

Manual guidance should strive to be, wherever possible, active. Active techniques possess a greater number of plastic code elements than do passive techniques. Active techniques will facilitate the adaptive response and increase the eventuality that change will be maintained long after the cessation of treatment. However, this principle should not be applied too rigidly in treatment. It has been shown that a mixture of active and passive movement guidance does contribute

to the improvement of motor skills,[159] and furthermore, some patients may be too disabled actively to use their bodies. In this situation, rehabilitation has to start with passive techniques. As soon as the patient is showing an improved ability in active movement, the treatment should shift towards the use of active techniques.

DYNAMIC AND STATIC TECHNIQUES

Afferent recruitment

This area has been explored above. In essence, dynamic manual events recruit and activate a larger array of mechanoreceptors and increase their overall firing rate, which leads to an increased barrage of proprioceptive feedback on the CNS.

Proprioceptive acuity

When a subject's finger is held in static position, it seems that either passive–static or active–static makes very little contribution to proprioceptive acuity.[61,75] These two situations seem to be inferior to active–dynamic and passive–dynamic events, the awareness of joint movement increasing only when dynamic events take place (see Fig. 9.11 above). This was also demonstrated during direct recording of neurons in the sensory cortex of an awake animal. Of the 227 neurons affected by joint movement, 196 responded to dynamic joint movement, whilst only 31 responded to static joint positions, usually at extreme joint ranges.[22]

The rate at which a limb is being moved is also important in treatment. Proprioceptive acuity during slow, low-amplitude passive movement can be so poor that, in one study, subjects found it difficult to identify whether the joint was moving into flexion or extension.[160] On many occasions, their judgement of the direction of joint movement related to previous movements. Sometimes, the subjects incorrectly identified movement at the elbow when the elbow remained immobile, and vice versa. The awareness of joint position is markedly increased during rapid passive movement.[72] However, if movement is too rapid, it will also tend to reduce acuity.[3] The amplitude of joint movement also plays an important role in producing changes in the temporal afferent volley and subsequently joint acuity. Generally, large-amplitude movements produce greater afferent volley and increase acuity compared with low-amplitude movement. However, amplitude of movement is closely linked to rate of movement. In general, a greater proprioceptive response is achieved with more rapid and larger-amplitude movements (except when these elements are exaggerated into any extreme, Fig. 9.13).

Another interesting finding in these experiments has been that when dynamic motion (whether active or passive), is terminated there is a gradual deterioration in proprioceptive acuity, which tapers off after about 15 seconds. This has been attributed to the adaptation time of dynamic joint and spindle afferents, which also occurs over a period of 15 seconds.

Learning and transfer

Normal motor learning processes are almost exclusively dynamic rather than static (see

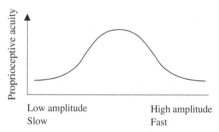

Figure 9.13 The amplitude and velocity of the joint will affect proprioceptive acuity. Acuity generally reduces at both extremes.

Fig. 9.11 above). In learning to use a screwdriver, it is not enough to hold it in your hand: dynamic patterns of muscle activity must be initiated in order for the skill to be memorized. Because transfer between motor tasks is fairly specific, static techniques may not transfer well to dynamic movement in daily activities. Manual technique should imitate this natural form of encoding of motor acts, suggesting that rehabilitation should be a dynamic event.

In a pilot study of balance ability in healthy subjects, we were able to demonstrate the effectiveness of active, passive, dynamic and static techniques on motor learning.[161] Subjects were tested for their balancing ability before and after four modes of manual intervention: massage of the whole lower limb for 3 minutes (passive–static); knee oscillation at full flexion for 3 minutes (passive–dynamic); eight cycles of hip and knee extension from 90° to straight leg against resistance (active–dynamic); and while standing, balance being challenged by the therapist, gently pushing the subject off balance in different directions (active–dynamic but with a strong transfer element) (see Fig. 9.7 above). All techniques except the passive–static significantly improved balancing ability. The active technique with the transfer element was most effective, then, in descending order, active–dynamic, passive–dynamic and passive–static techniques. Both active techniques were significantly more effective than were the passive techniques. This study also highlights the importance of transfer as a part of treatment. For example, if walking is rehabilitated, movement that imitates the neuromuscular patterns of walking may transfer well to daily functional use of the limb.[130,132,162]

10

Manual guidance in the treatment of dysfunction and damage in the motor system

This section looks at the neural processes associated with dysfunction in the motor system and their rehabilitation by manual therapy. Dysfunction in the motor system can arise under different conditions:

1. The intact nervous system:
   a. Abnormal postural and movement patterns.
   b. neuromuscular dysfunction following musculoskeletal injury.
2. The damaged nervous system:
   a. Incomplete development of the motor programme due to damage, before maturation in the young.
   b. Central damage to the nervous system, in adult life, after the motor system has functionally matured.

THE INTACT NERVOUS SYSTEM

ABNORMAL POSTURAL AND MOVEMENT PATTERNS

The motor system has an impressive capacity to learn and store a large selection of motor programmes throughout life. Most often, this storage is useful and contributes positively to the individual's motor activities. However, this learning capacity can act as a double-edged sword: from time to time non-productive motor activity can be picked up by the system, stored and used in physical situations where it is of no use to the performance of the motor task.

An example of such abnormal activity is tensing the neck and shoulder muscles during typing. Tensing the shoulders has no functional use and usually causes fatigue and discomfort. In time and with repetition, this pattern will be stored as part of the programme for typing. In such a case, the aim of the treatment is to promote normal function. This can be done by teaching the individual to relax the shoulders during various physical activities or advising the patient about the optimum sitting posture and correct patterns of movement. By cognition and re-experiencing, this pattern will eventually become the dominant motor activity used during typing (Fig. 10.1).

I often use this simple approach in treating chronic neck and shoulder conditions. While the patient is writing or typing, I use verbal and manual feedback in guiding the patient to relax while working. Manually, I gently guide the shoulders and neck into an 'optimal' posture. Verbal feedback is used to inform patients how

well they are relaxing their muscles. Following treatment, the patient is encouraged to transfer the treatment experience to the work situation in order to facilitate the learning process.

Many musculoskeletal injuries are probably related to abnormal movement patterns that are imposed on the musculoskeletal system, producing structural damage. This can be seen in abnormal movement patterns in sporting activities (e.g. abnormal patterns of serving in tennis, resulting in tennis elbow or shoulder damage) and work activities (e.g. abnormal patterns of typing, resulting in repetitive strain injuries). This does not exclude acute injuries, in which an extreme movement pattern results in major structural damage, such as a wrong pattern of bending leading to disc herniation. Tissue repair may be impeded by movement repeated in the pattern of the original injury. For a successful treatment outcome, the therapist has to identify the noxious movement and guide the patient into the correct pattern. This reduces the potential for structural damage and helps to conserve physical energy in daily living. Failing to do this will result in unsuccessful and transient improvement as the patient is continuously being injured by repetition of the noxious movement.

NEUROMUSCULAR DYSFUNCTION FOLLOWING MUSCULOSKELETAL INJURY

A common sequel to musculoskeletal injury is neuromuscular changes (Fig. 10.2) arising from several sources:

- changes in proprioception by altered activity of mechanoreceptors
- inhibition from the joint afferents in conditions where there is direct damage to the joint
- altered motor patterns brought about by psychomotor responses
- reflex responses to pain.

This chapter will discuss the underlying physiological mechanisms and possible treatment modalities that may help to reverse these changes. Pain mechanisms are discussed in all three Sections of the book.

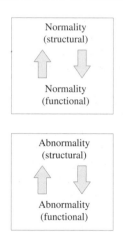

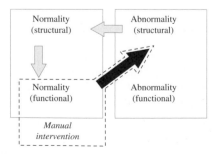

Figure 10.1 The relationship between function and structure within the motor system.

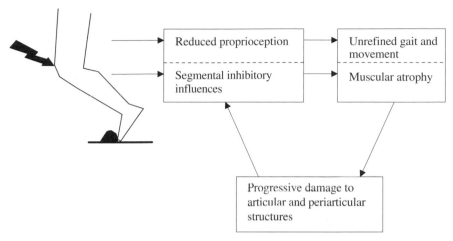

Figure 10.2 A possible mechanism of progressive joint damage.

Proprioceptive changes following injury

Injuries to muscles and joints may lead to loss of proprioception from the affected area, producing functional (rather than structural) instability.[141,162–166] In this condition, the supporting structures of the joint may be intact, but there is during movement abnormal neuromuscular activity at the joint, which results in instability. For example, in the ankle joint, functional instability is often seen when the ankle 'gives way' during walking. In this condition, passive examination of the ankle may not reveal any structural damage to account for this instability.

Proprioceptive losses following injury have been shown to occur in the spine, knee, ankle and temporomandibular joint.[141,167–170] Proprioceptive loss in the long term is believed to contribute to progressive degenerative joint disease and muscular atrophy.[163,164] In these conditions, the motor system has lost an important source of feedback for the refinement of movement. This may result in abnormal gait patterns, producing abnormal mechanical stress on joint structures.

Reduced proprioception has been reported following lower back injuries.[168] This could potentially alter normal neuromuscular activity at the spinal joints and contribute to further spinal damage and progressive degenerative changes. Similarly, reduced proprioception has been reported in knee joints following injury, repair, surgical intervention and degenerative joint disease.[171,172] Subjects with cruciate ligament damage have been shown to have reduced proprioceptive acuity in the knee.[167] Following surgical repair of the cruciate ligaments, patients who returned to normal sporting activity were found to be dependent on the degree of proprioceptive acuity rather than on the stability of the knee or the quality of the surgical repair.[173]

The effects of proprioceptive deficit on motor activity may take time to develop, which may suggest a negatively acting neuroplastic process. When assessing postural steadiness 3 weeks after lateral ligament injury of the ankle, only negligible changes in steadiness have taken place. However, after 9 months, the balance deficit can be observed in 61% of subjects.[174]

Proposed mechanisms of reduced proprioception

The mechanisms underlying reduction of proprioception are not fully understood. Some proposed mechanisms are:

- local chemical changes at the receptor site
- damage to the receptor or its axon
- damage and structural changes in the tissue in which the receptor is embedded.

Local chemical changes at the receptor site

Changes in the receptor's chemical environment, which may be brought about by ischaemic or inflammatory events, may affect its sensitivity. Reduced proprioception has been observed in muscle fatigue produced by high-intensity exercise.[175,176] It has been suggested that muscle afferents are affected by the build-up of metabolic byproducts, which may lead to diminished proprioception.[177] The mechanism for this altered sensitivity is stimulation of group III and IV afferents from the muscle (mainly pain afferents). These induce excitation of the intrafusal motor-neurons, with a subsequent alteration in sensitivity of the spindle afferents.[177] In joint damage, inflammatory byproducts sensitize the group III and IV afferents.

Damage to the receptor or its axon

Physical trauma can affect the receptors and their axons directly. The articular receptors and their axons have a lower tensile strength than do the collagen fibres in which they are embedded.[141] So injury to the capsule and ligaments will damage the receptors embedded in these tissues. Similarly, in direct trauma to muscle, the spindles and their innervation may be damaged, leading to a reduction in and altered pattern of proprioception. If the parent muscle is denervated and renervated, the spindle afferents will redevelop. This is an adaptive process that is highly dependent on the contractile activity of the extrafusal fibres.[178,179]

Damage and structural changes in the tissue in which the receptor is embedded

Any structural changes in the parent tissue may lead to atrophy of the receptor and changes in its ability to detect movement. For example, in muscle, immobilization or damage can lead to spindle atrophy. These structural changes have been shown to alter the sensitivity and firing rate of spindle afferents during passive stretching.[180]

Adhesions and tears of the parent tissue will probably also alter the mechanical ability of the receptor to detect movement. For example, local capsular adhesion around the receptor can potentially reduce the receptor's ability to detect the normal range of movement.

Reflexogenic effects of musculoskeletal injury

Compounding functional instability is the loss of muscle force and the wasting that are often seen following joint injury. It has been demonstrated that this reduction in voluntary activation is mediated by joint afferents. The alteration in the afferent pattern from the damaged area may result in the initiation of central processes that inhibit the motorneurons supplying the affected muscle (rather than the joint afferents 'switching off' the motorneurons directly).[66] The main group of afferents believed to produce this inhibition are group III mechanoreceptors and group IV nociceptors. However, this inhibitory state can be seen even in damaged, pain-free joints, which suggests that this process can be solely mediated by group III afferents.

Arthrogenic inhibition has been observed during knee effusion and inflammation, resulting in quadriceps weakness and wasting.[181–185] In a chronically damaged knee, this inhibition has been shown to be present even without joint effusion or inflammation.[164] Arthrogenic inhibition has also been observed in the elbow joint,[187] and similar processes probably take place in the spinal facet joints following injury.

Psychomotor response to injury

Often musculoskeletal injuries are associated with psychological processes related to the body-self and body-image (see Section 3). Psychomotor processes can alter the pattern of muscle recruitment at a local level and bring about postural compensations affecting the whole body. For example, a feeling of insecurity about using the damaged area and evasive behaviour as a result of pain can profoundly alter normal patterns of movement. These situations can lead to plastic neuromuscular changes, one of which can be disuse muscle weakness.

Reducing pain and increasing strength will change the evasive behaviour, promote normal neuro-muscular activity and a positive change in body-image. Methods for reducing pain and rehabilitating the neuro-muscular link are discussed throughout the book. Working with psychological processes such as body-image are discussed in Section 3.

Manual rehabilitation of musculoskeletal injuries

In the two conditions described above, the rehabilitation approach aims to achieve the following objectives:

- to override inhibitory influences and improve voluntary activation
- to improve proprioception
- to reduce pain.

The management of pain at the neurological level is discussed in Chapter 12.

Override inhibitory influences and improve voluntary activation

There are no current studies of the effect of manual therapy on arthrogenic inhibition. Some indications of the form of manipulation can be derived from studies of the effect of joint aspiration on arthrogenic inhibition. In the acutely effused joint, arthrogenic inhibition has been shown to be reduced by needle aspiration. Manually, this may be achieved by rhythmic passive joint movement, as described in Section 1.

Another indication of the form of manipulation is derived from studies of the effect of exercise on arthrogenic inhibition.[187,188] Subjects with anterior cruciate ligament damage of the knee usually display the characteristic arthrogenic inhibitory pattern. During movement into extension, at angle of about 40°, there is an observable decrease in quadriceps force and EMG activity (Fig. 10.3). This reduction in activity is compensated by an increase in hamstring activity. In trained individuals with similar damage, this inhibitory pattern is seen in EMG activity but not in force of contraction, a similar force to that of healthy subjects being displayed. It seems that physical training has normalized the neuromuscular activity regardless of background inhibition. This has been shown also to

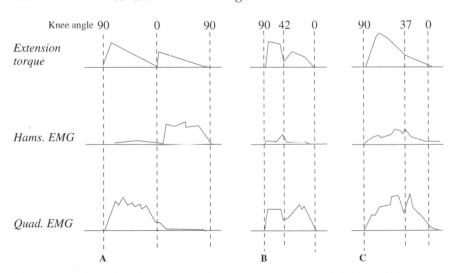

Figure 10.3 Extension torque and EMG activity of the hamstrings and quadriceps muscles. (A) Normal subjects. (B) Subjects with anterior cruciate damage. There is reduced force production at 42° of knee extension, with reduced hamstring activity and a compensatory increase in quadriceps activity. (C) Subjects with cruciate damage but with tight hamstrings. There is no failure in extension torque, although there is EMG activity of the hamstrings and quadriceps similar to that seen in (B). Comparable findings were found in subjects who exercised regularly. (After Solomonow et al 1987 with permission.[186])

occur in functional instability of the ankle: treatment by coordination exercise virtually eliminates the symptoms of instability.[141] Similarly, in patients with early osteoarthritis of the knees, exercise rehabilitation has been shown to improve voluntary activation.[164] In both of these examples, the overriding influences are probably derived from higher centres within the motor system, which highlights the importance of volition in overcoming the inhibitory state. These studies indicate that active techniques would be effective in overriding the inhibitory process. This is supported by studies demonstrating that active–dynamic rather than active–static techniques (see the previous section on manual guidance and motor abilities) have a greater overriding influence on arthrogenic inhibition.[186] It should be noted that patients with severe damage to the joint and without surgical repair may not respond as well to neuromuscular rehabilitation.

Improve proprioception

Techniques that could enhance proprioception must contain two important functional elements:

1. They must be able to maximally stimulate the different groups of mechanoreceptors from and around the damaged area.
2. They must be able to simulate the normal sensory and motor patterns.

Of the different modes of manual techniques, only one group of techniques – active–dynamic – can successfully fulfil these two requirements. These will maximally increase both the temporal and spatial afferent volley, as well as providing the continuous matching of the sensory feedback to ongoing motor processes.

Manual implications

It can be concluded that active modes of manipulation will be most effective in reversing some of the neurogenic changes following musculoskeletal injury. Initially, low-force active–dynamic techniques can be used, with progressive increases in force. The increase in force has to be graded against various factors such as tensile strength of the healing joint, pain levels, inflammation and improvement in neuromuscular activity. In my own clinical experience, adverse reactions can occur if active techniques are introduced too early, before improvements in repair have taken place. Once pain is reduced and the patient is able to weight-bear on the injured leg, balancing and whole body movements should be encouraged.[141,147] The use of dynamic techniques should be within the spectrum of abilities, and they should be matched to the patient's movement needs in daily and leisure activities. If active techniques are used, the patient should not be allowed to become fatigued or develop pain as this could transiently reduce proprioception.[174,175] The rehabilitation of musculoskeletal injuries is summarized in Fig. 10.4.

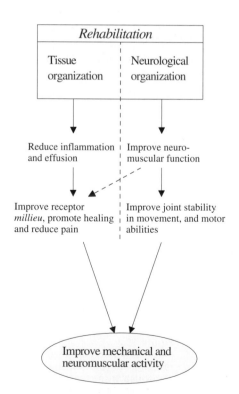

Figure 10.4   Aims of manual treatment in the rehabilitation of joint injury.

THE DAMAGED NERVOUS SYSTEM

INCOMPLETE DEVELOPMENT OF THE MOTOR PROGRAMME DUE TO DAMAGE BEFORE MATURATION IN THE YOUNG, AND LOSS OF MOTOR FUNCTION IN ADULT LIFE AFTER THE MOTOR PROGRAMME HAS MATURED

Rehabilitation of neuromuscular function in the young and the adult is essentially similar with respect to the use of motor abilities. However, there are some differences between the adult's and the child's motor system (Fig. 10.5), one principle being that the adult has completed motor development, and most newly learned movements are thus made up of previous experiences (see above). In the young, motor acts are truly novel and are not composed of fragments of previous experiences. This means that the child has to learn the movement 'from scratch', implying a long rehabilitation process. Rehabilitation using sequential development principles may be useful for the disabled child, but this type of rehabilitation is probably unnecessary in the adult. Interestingly, within my circle of friends, two different parents have told me that one of their children (children without any motor disability) did not follow the normal sequence of motor development. For example, one child never crawled, progressing from lying to sitting to walking. This raises the question of whether the full sequence is essential for rehabilitation.

Central damage to the motor system can result in complex and widely varying functional disabilities. A description of all the potential damages and functional changes is outside the scope of this book, and the reader should refer to more detailed texts. Carpenter's analogy of the motor system as a military hierarchy is useful for understanding central motor damage and rehabilitation.[53] In this model, the higher centres are the generals: the decision-making ranks. The spinal centres or lower centres are the soldiers, who execute the commands from the higher centre. If one of the soldiers, or a group of soldiers, is injured, it will only affect the position that they are holding, without necessarily affecting other parts of the hierarchy. An example of this is peripheral nerve injury.

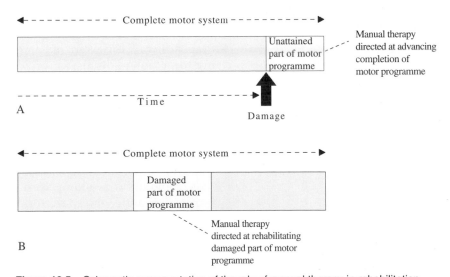

Figure 10.5 Schematic representation of the role of manual therapy in rehabilitation. (A) Rehabilitation in the young before the completion of motor programme development. (B) Rehabilitation aims in the treatment of the adult once the motor programme has been fully developed.

However, if the headquarters are hit and some of the generals are injured or killed, the downflow of command will be disrupted. Initially, the soldiers may be unaffected by this change and will continue to perform their appointed tasks. In time, and without an overview of the battlefield, their assessment of their role will disintegrate and they will initiate their own activity, firing without any overall plan. An example of this is spasticity, in which, following loss of higher centre control, spinal centres will initiate their own motor activity (Fig. 10.6). This motor dysfunction is usually unrelated to the movement goal of the individual.

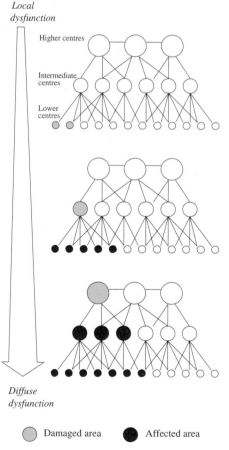

Figure 10.6   The extent of disability is related to the level and size of damage within the motor system. Although damage is portrayed in this diagram as occurring on a vertical expansion, it can also occur on a lateral expansion, in which centres lateral to the damage are affected.

The loss of higher centre control is commonly manifested in muscles as either hyper- or hypo-activity. Hyperactivity is the release of spinal centres from the inhibitory control of higher centres and is often manifested as spasticity.[188] Hypoactivity is due to reduced motor drive to muscles, which results in loss of muscle force and flaccidity. Both these conditions can be viewed functionally as miscommunication between the different motor centres (or discontinuity in structural terms). Depending on the localization and magnitude of the damage, abilities and skills will also be affected.

Following damage to the higher motor centres, the segmental influence of mechanoreceptors may become exaggerated, resulting in abnormal muscle activity, for example the clasp-knife reflex or lead pipe reflex. This will impede the individual's ability to perform normal physical activity, as any attempt to produce movement will be overrun by abnormal muscle activity.

REHABILITATION OF CENTRAL MOTOR DAMAGE

If the damage in the central nervous system causes discontinuity and miscommunication, rehabilitation can be seen as the drive to restore these linkages. This relies on neuroplasticity and the regenerative capacity of neural tissue (depending on the extent of damage). Incorporating previously discussed principles of motor learning and guidance, the treatment aims can be broken down into a sequence that can simplify the rehabilitation programme, for example:

- *Aim 1*: Identify the discrepancy between the potential and the actual motor performance of the patient, for example, how 'far' the patient is from normal walking (see also Fig. 7.2).
- *Aim 2*: Identify the source of discrepancy: For example, balance is saved, but there is hypertonia of leg muscles.
- *Aim 3*: Approximate the discrepancy by rehabilitation. For example, if balance is affected, work with balance abilities, etc. (see the text above on manual guidance and motor abilities).

- *Aim 4*: If the approximation process is impeded by spasticity, techniques to inhibit the overactive centres should be used. Once spasticity is reduced, the approximation process is then immediately continued.
- *Aim 5*: Reduce muscle and connective tissue shortening. Use stretching techniques to elongate shortened tissue (as discussed in Ch. 3). If the patient has a loss of motor drive (i.e. muscle weakness), passive stretching techniques (the patient will be unable to produce the contraction force necessary for active stretching) should initially be employed.
- *Aim 6*: Pain relief. Severe musculoskeletal pain can accompany motor disability. Passive techniques, such as soft-tissue massage and articulation, should be used for pain management (see also Chs 4 and 5).

Reducing spasticity

There are numerous methods of reducing muscle spasticity (probably as many as there are practitioners). One must remember that promoting normal functional movement rather than reducing spasticity, is the ultimate goal of rehabilitation. Of the methods of reducing spasticity, probably the most important are those promoting conscious relaxation and cognitive/volitional movement. These techniques encourage continuity, communication and control within the whole motor system. Some of these techniques are described below.

Motor relaxation. Guidance is used to direct the patient in relaxing the hyperactive muscles. Conscious inhibition encourages connectivity and control between the higher and lower motor centres.

Motor facilitation. Volition involves the potent influences of the higher motor centres, which may override the abnormal motor activity initiated by lower centres. In this method, the patient is encouraged to use the hyperactive muscles in a functional pattern (using abilities, see Ch. 9). Voluntary muscle activity also implies connectivity and control between the different motor centres. Spasticity may mask an underlying loss of muscle force (personal observation). Guidance in different force abilities can be used to increase muscle strength.

Agonist/antagonist (central) reciprocal activation (rather than peripheral reciprocal inhibition). Slow movement utilizing the agonist may help to reduce antagonist activity.

Active trunk, neck or limb rotation. Neck may reduce hyperactivity in the movement limb. 'Constructive fiddling' with different positions may reveal inhibitory patterns. This pattern may not be constant (reproducible) in the same patient and may change from one patient to another.

Slow stretch of agonists. This may reduce the hyperactivity in the stretched muscle.

11

Muscle tone and motor tone

One contentious area in manual therapy is that of muscle tone. There is a general belief that muscles have a sustained, low-level neurological 'tone' even when the individual is resting, and that some forms of manipulation can reduce persistent abnormal tone. Below, we will consider normal and abnormal muscle tone and how manipulation can help to bring about changes in tone.

In normal circumstances, changes in tone can be observed during muscle activity and relaxation. Muscle tissue is seen to have two 'existential' states:

1. Passive state: In its resting state, the muscle has no internal contractile activity and responds to external mechanical stimuli as would other innate structures such as ligaments. When palpated, the muscle may feel tight or soft, and in this passive state the muscle is said to have mechanical tone. This type of tone will be termed *muscle tone*.

2. Active state: The active state occurs when a muscle is contracting in response to a command from the motor system. When palpated, the muscle will show varying degrees of tightness, depending on the force of contraction. Although there is an actual structural change in the muscle and a rise in mechanical tone (as in muscle tone), the source of this tone is neurological. This active state of the muscle is termed *motor tone*.

The differences created by motor and muscle tone can be readily palpated in normal muscle. If one rests the forearm, fully relaxed, on a table (with the elbow flexed to 90°) and palpates the relaxed biceps, it will feel like a balloon filled with gel. This is the muscle's resting tone (there being no motor activity in the muscle). Fully straightening the arm (letting it hang by the side fully relaxed), will passively elongate the biceps muscle, which, when palpated, will feel more rigid. It will no longer feel like a bag of gel, but more like a bag filled with gel and strands of spaghetti. The increase in stiffness is purely an internal mechanical event resulting from passive elongation of muscle fibres, fascia and other connective tissue elements, and an increase in intramuscular pressure. There is still no neurological motor tone in the muscle. If one actively flexes the elbow to 90° and palpates the muscle, it will feel hard and rubbery. This is the result of an increase in intramuscular pressure brought about by the active contraction of the muscle cells in response to a motor command. If the muscle is fully relaxed, it will again feel flaccid.

MUSCLE TONE

Muscle tone is created by the biomechanical elements in the muscle. This tone is a mixture of tension in the fascia and connective tissue elements and intramuscular fluid pressure. In normal individuals, there is no neurological (motor) tone in skeletal muscles during rest.[142] This has an important biological logic. Muscle activity is energy consuming; it would be energetically wasteful to maintain muscle activity during rest, and energy conservation is an important principle in most human activities.[188] Some believe that sustained muscle tone is necessary for the maintenance of blood flow in resting muscle. However, blood flow in resting muscle is maintained by pulsatile arteriolar activity. The pulsations are interrupted during muscle contraction.[189] Continuous contraction during rest would therefore reduce the flow to the muscle rather than increase it.[190-194]

MOTOR TONE

Motor tone is initiated by the motor system to produce purposeful movement and posture.

Some motor tone will be transient (phasic), such as that during lifting or correcting the balance when falling. Other activity is more sustained (tonic), for example that of postural muscles in keeping the body upright. When an individual lies down and relaxes, both the phasic and the tonic muscles are neurologically silent.[157,195,196]

In our 'class lab', we often demonstrate the neurological silence of muscle during rest. Students are asked to lie fully relaxed while EMG recordings are taken from different muscles and compared with EMG readings taken from skin overlying bone (i.e. with no muscle underneath). Providing the subjects are fully relaxed, there is no evidence of motor tone. The EMG trace taken over the bone is no different from that taken from a relaxed muscle. Similar EMG activity can be observed in painful muscular conditions such as muscle fatigue (subjects volunteer to exercise a muscle until pain and fatigue develop), acute or chronic back pain or muscular injury (in each class there are quite a few of these). When the subjects are resting, the EMG trace shows no neurological activity even when there are reports of considerable muscle pain and a palpable raised muscle tone.

Another fact in support of the principle of a lack of resting motor tone comes from the extensive studies cited throughout this section on motorneuron excitability.[99,100,102-104,107] Because there is no motor tone in normal resting muscle, the only possibility for observing the state of the motor system is by stimulating the motorneurons; i.e. motor control rather than the muscle itself is studied.

ABNORMAL MUSCLE AND MOTOR TONE

In normal circumstances, muscle has the functional flexibility to move from one state to another without any difficulty or residual problems. However, this flexibility can fail, for example as a result of overactivity of or damage to the motor system. There will then be changes in both muscle and motor tone. For lack of a better term, this will be called 'abnormal tone', which can be defined as *tone that does not support functional movement and may outlast the activity that initiated it*. For example, during running, there will be an increase in both muscle and motor tone. Following the run, when the individual is resting, there may be a residual increase in intramuscular pressure that is mechanical in nature. This tone has outlasted the running and no longer supports it. Similarly, in neurological damage, the abnormal motor tone often gets in the way of normal purposeful movement, outlasts it and may extend into periods of rest.

ABNORMAL MUSCLE TONE

A rise in muscle tone is a common finding when palpating muscles. There are several mechanisms that can cause an increase in muscle tone (Fig. 11.1). Some are normal changes related to the length of the muscle (during rest) and some are due to local pathomechanical changes in the muscle:

- normal increase in tone in relaxed muscle:
  - positional influences: passive length changes in the muscle
  - transient fluid accumulation: such as in muscle following exercising
- Abnormal increase in tone in relaxed muscle:
  - prolonged fluid accumulation: due to impediment to flow, such as in compartment syndrome

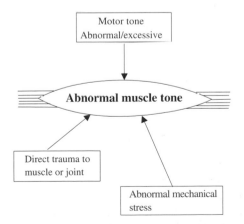

Figure 11.1 Possible mechanisms producing abnormal muscle tone.

- structural changes: These may be due to changes in the ratio of muscle tissue to connective tissue elements, or overall structural shortening of the muscle cell and connective tissue elements.

Positional influences

Normal changes in muscle tone owing to passive changes of position are only clinically important during the examination stage. If the muscle is palpated in its lengthened position, it will feel tight, giving the false impression that there is something wrong with it. Ideally, muscle tone should be evaluated when the joint lies in its resting angle and the muscle is neither too lax nor too tight.

Transient fluid accumulation

Increases in muscle tone following exercise are a common clinical finding. They are brought about by an increase of intramuscular pressure as a result of increased blood volume, transient fluid accumulation and oedema. In this situation, intermittent compression or rhythmic active pump techniques can be used to increase the flow through the muscle (see Ch. 5).[197]

Prolonged fluid accumulation

Long-term muscle activity and mechanical stress can lead to structural changes in the muscle that can lead to reduced flow through the muscle, resulting in hypoxia, oedema and cellular damage. This type of tone is commonly seen in muscle compartment syndrome. In this condition, the fascia surrounding the muscle constricts the natural swelling of the muscle and vascular flow during and following exercise.[198] This results in high intramuscular pressure, which impedes normal flow through the muscle. Compartment syndromes have been shown to occur in the leg muscles and, more recently, in spinal muscles.[199]

Different approaches can be used to treat long-term fluid accumulation. Passive pump techniques can facilitate flow away from the muscle (see Ch. 5). Active pump techniques may initially be less beneficial as they tend to cause an increase in intramuscular pressure, fatigue and pain. Longitudinal and cross-fibre soft-tissue stretches can be used to elongate and loosen the muscle's connective tissue envelope (see Ch. 4).

Structural changes

Prolonged muscle activity, especially with the muscle in the shortened position, will lead to changes in length of both the muscle cell and the connective tissue elements. The ratio of number and size of muscle cells to connective tissue elements within the muscle will also change with time. Manual techniques that could help re-elongate the muscle are longitudinal, cross-fibre stretching and active stretching techniques (see Section 1).

In musculoskeletal damage, the common palpable increase in resting tone is probably related to the structural, morphological changes in the muscle. These are *biomechanical changes* rather than changes in motor tone.

ABNORMAL MOTOR TONE

Spontaneous non-purposeful motor activity in muscles can be seen in several conditions:

- damage to the motor system
- psychological stress
- protective muscle activity following injury.

Damage to the motor system

Central motor damage will often result in spontaneous motor tone. This is seen in such diverse neurological conditions as stroke, spasticity, cerebral palsy and Parkinson's disease. In these conditions, the muscle may be in a tonic state, twitching or contracting in any other non-purposeful way. Some of the techniques used for reducing abnormal motor tone have been described in this section.

Neurological pathologies such as multiple sclerosis can manifest as a slow, insidious onset of abnormal muscular activity. In fully relaxed individuals not suffering from stress and anxiety, who have no difficulty in relaxing and who are not in severe pain, abnormal non-purposeful muscle contraction may be an early sign of central nervous system pathology.

Psychological stress

Emotional stress, anxiety and arousal are some of the psychological states that will influence general motor tone.[142] This change in tone is not associated with pathology of the motor system.

During treatment, most individuals can relax and reduce their level of muscle tension. However, on rare occasions, some individuals find it difficult to 'let go' and fully relax.[142] This will manifest itself as a general increase in motor tone. In treating motor tone of psychological origin, the use of expressive manipulation rather than a mechanistic approach is advocated. Differences between expressive and instrumental manipulation are discussed in detail in Section 3.

Protective muscle activity following injury

Sustained motor tone is often seen following musculoskeletal injury. This is a protective mechanism used to splint the damage or prevent use of the injured area. Depending on the severity of the injury, patients are usually able to relax their muscles fully when positioned in a non-painful, non-stressful position, protective contractions usually returning when they move back to a painful position. In these conditions, treatment should be directed at the cause rather than its motor component, i.e. reducing inflammation and pain and facilitating repair.

Loss of motor tone

There are several conditions in which motor tone to the muscle is reduced or totally abolished. In central nervous system damage and peripheral nerve injury, motor tone can be reduced, resulting in flaccid muscle. In both conditions, the return of motor tone depends on the quality of repair. Another common condition in which motor tone is reduced is following joint injury (arthrogenic inhibition). This has been discussed above.

IDENTIFYING CAUSE AND OUTCOME IN MUSCLE AND MOTOR TONE CONDITIONS

Both causes and outcomes of abnormal muscle and motor tone must be identified and treated; failure to do so may provide only a partial solution to the patient's condition.

In stress-related conditions in which there are muscle tone changes and pain, treatment should be directed towards reducing arousal (cause) as well as working on long-term structural changes to the muscle (outcome). In central motor damage, the overall direction of the treatment is toward rehabilitating the motor system (cause), but any structural changes (outcome) that may be as a result of abnormal motor tone should also be addressed. Stressful and irregular use of the muscle could result in compartment syndrome, whose treatment should aim to identify the cause (abnormal use) as well as its outcome (increased mechanical tension in the muscle's compartment). In conditions marked by pain with protective muscle contraction, the aim is to reduce inflammation and pain (cause). This eventually will lead to a normalization of motor tone (outcome). The causes and treatment aims of abnormal muscle and motor tone are summarized in Figure 11.2.

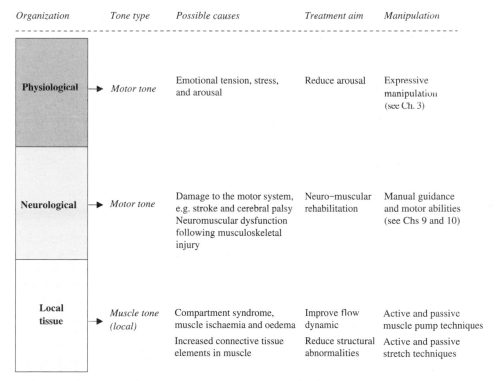

Organization	Tone type	Possible causes	Treatment aim	Manipulation
Physiological	*Motor tone*	Emotional tension, stress, and arousal	Reduce arousal	Expressive manipulation (see Ch. 3)
Neurological	*Motor tone*	Damage to the motor system, e.g. stroke and cerebral palsy Neuromuscular dysfunction following musculoskeletal injury	Neuro–muscular rehabilitation	Manual guidance and motor abilities (see Chs 9 and 10)
Local tissue	*Muscle tone (local)*	Compartment syndrome, muscle ischaemia and oedema	Improve flow dynamic	Active and passive muscle pump techniques
		Increased connective tissue elements in muscle	Reduce structural abnormalities	Active and passive stretch techniques

Figure 11.2 Abnormal muscle tone and motor tone can be of different origin.

12

Pain relief by manipulation– neurological mechanisms

This chapter examines the possible neurological mechanisms attributed to pain reduction during manipulation. Here, too, there will be little discussion of anatomy, most of the information relating to the functional aspects of pain.

RECEPTORS, PATHWAYS AND CENTRAL PROCESSING

Section 1 discussed how, during inflammation, mechanical, chemical and thermal irritation excites the local pain-conveying receptors.[199] Although free nerve endings have been implicated as the specialized receptors for conveying noxious stimuli (and therefore the sensation of pain), other receptors such as mechanoreceptors from the skin, muscles and joints can also contribute to the sensation of pain.[200] The more specialized pain-conveying nerve fibres are called 'nociceptors'; however, they can also convey other sensory modalities such as temperature, and mechanical stimuli such as tactile and movement stimuli.[200,201] Thus, the complex pattern of pain is probably evoked by the stimulation of several types of receptor simultaneously. Within the nervous system, there is no single centre that subserves the discriminative, cognitive and motivational dimensions of pain.[200] Pain experience involves the operation of various subsystems and pathways and is not determined exclusively by any one of them.[200] The same is true with pain-conveying pathways: some also convey other sensory information. The fact that pain is not a structural entity within the nervous system highlights the importance of function rather than (at a neurological level) structure in pain management.

NEUROFUNCTIONAL ASPECTS OF PAIN: POSSIBLE IMPLICATIONS FOR MANIPULATION

There are several functional aspects of pain that may be affected by different forms of manipulation. Understanding these neurological mechanisms may help the therapist in two ways:

- reducing pain by manipulation (manual analgesia)
- reducing the potential for adverse reactions.

MANIPULATION-INDUCED ANALGESIA

A common clinical finding is that immediate pain relief can occur during various manual techniques. In some conditions, pain may be reduced by manual techniques such as stroking of the skin, deep kneading, articulation and muscle contraction.

Gating of sensory activity

One possible explanation for manually induced analgesia may be related to a neurological process called sensory gating. In sensory gating, the processing and perception of one sensory modality may be reduced by a concomitant stimulation of another. For example, during muscle contraction, normal and noxious sensory sensation from the skin may be reduced.[202] This is also shown when electrical, tactile and vibrational (test) stimuli are applied to the skin during different limb activities (gating stimulus).[203–209] Similarly, the perception of certain types of noxious stimulus applied to the skin may be reduced during active[210] and passive[203] movement, and vibration of the skin.[211] In one study, a specialized ring-shaped vibrator was used to observe the effect of vibration on pain perception during noxious stimulation of the skin. During vibration, the noxious stimulus was applied to the skin through the centre of the vibrator ring. When vibration and the noxious stimulus were applied simultaneously, the subjects perceived a lower intensity and poorer localization of the pain. Once the vibrator was switched off, the intensity of pain rose to its previbration level.[211] This change in pain perception is also seen when the vibrator is not applied to the site of injury (although being applied not too far away from it). This implies that the changes in pain level are not due to the local effects of the vibrator on inflammatory mechanism but to modulation of neurological activity. It should be noted that, during sensory gating, the perception of test stimulus is never totally abolished but is usually slightly reduced.[212–215]

Melzack[216] describes these gating mechanisms as 'hyperstimulation analgesia' and suggests that therapeutic modalities such as transcutaneous electric stimulation, acupuncture and even counterirritation methods (for example, mustard plasters, ice packs or blistering agents) can produce pain relief by sensory gating.

Neurophysiological mechanisms in gating

As previously discussed, the central nervous system disregards much of the incoming sensory activity as being irrelevant, whilst being able to attend selectively to information that is deemed important.[48] Sensory gating is not limited to conscious activity but occurs automatically at lower levels within the nervous system (Fig. 12.1). These processes probably share common neurological mechanisms but differ in their complexity. Melzack & Wall proposed that, within the nervous system, there are mechanisms able to increase or decrease the flow of impulses from peripheral nerves to the central nervous system. These mechanisms act like a gate to sensory information.[217] Large-diameter nerve fibres, such as those from mechanoreceptors,[200] close the gate and contribute to pain relief, whilst small-diameter fibres, for example those from nociceptors,[200] open the gate, increasing the pain sensation.[217] This modulation of afferent activity

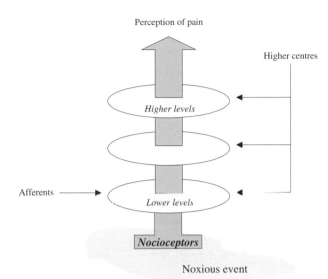

Perception of pain

Higher centres

Higher levels

Lower levels

Afferents

Nociceptors

Noxious event

Figure 12.1   Noxious sensory activity can be gated by descending influences from the higher centres or by non-nociceptor afferents in the vicinity of the irritation. Gating from higher centres can take place at different levels along the ascending pathway. Gating by afferents probably takes place at lower levels within the spinal cord.

may happen at different levels within the nervous system as the sensory information is conveyed centrally to higher centres. Sensory gating has been demonstrated within the spinal cord. When a recording electrode is inserted into an animal's dorsal horn, noxious stimulation of the skin will produce a distinct firing pattern from the dorsal horn neuron.[211] If vibration and a noxious stimulus are applied simultaneously, the vibration-induced firing pattern tends to alter the firing pattern of the noxious stimuli.

Another gating mechanism originates in higher centres and has descending influences on sensory activity (Fig. 12.1).[218–221] Gating by higher motor centres can be demonstrated, for example, during active movement. The perception of sensations from the skin tends to reduce just before active movement is initiated (surprisingly, this also occurs during passive movement).[204,222] This also occurs *during* active movement. It is estimated that the motor command plays only a minor role in sensory gating in comparison with the gating produced from the periphery.[203,210] However, other non-motor higher centres are more potent modulators of afferent activity. This

has been demonstrated by direct stimulation of various brain centres, during which pain was totally abolished for between many hours and many months.[219] The influences of higher centres and psychological processes on the perception of pain are further discussed in Section 3.

Manual gating

Gating processes imply that some manual techniques could be used to reduce pain sensation (Fig. 12.2). Some indication of the form of manipulation that could interrupt the pain pattern can be derived from such diverse sources as studies of phantom pain. After World War II, doctors found that many amputees with painful neuromas or phantom limb pain relieved their discomfort by drumming their fingers over the tender area of the stump (sometimes using mallets instead).[223] Other studies have demonstrated that a vibratory stimulus can reduce both acute and chronic pain in conditions where other treatment modalities have failed.[212–215] In many of these studies, pain relief outlasts the duration of the stimulus.[223,224] Sensory gating can often be seen in normal evasive behaviour to pain: stroking and rubbing of the skin over an area of injury.[225] In this situation, the individual is using a tactile gating stimulus to reduce the pain sensation.

In the studies described so far, the mechanical events producing the reduction in pain perception are almost always dynamic in character, for example active or passive movement and vibration of the skin. This implies that pain may be maximally gated by dynamic rather than static manual events. In general, although not always, active movement produces greater sensory gating than does passive movement.[203,206,207] This ties in well with the earlier description of proprioceptors and the expected increase in afferent activity during active and dynamic techniques compared with static techniques (see Ch. 8). Several forms of manipulation can fit these criteria (Table 12.1):

- percussive, massage and vibratory techniques[226]

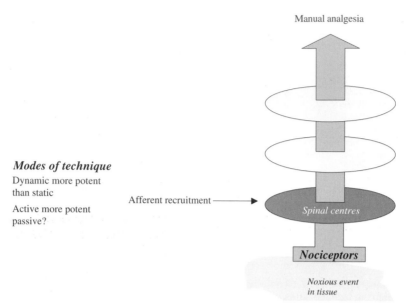

Modes of technique

Dynamic more potent
than static

Active more potent
passive?

Afferent recruitment ⟶

Manual analgesia

Spinal centres

Nociceptors

*Noxious event
in tissue*

Figure 12.2 Manual analgesia may occur by the activation of mechanoreceptors acting to gate nociception during different forms of manipulation.

- passive joint oscillation and articulation[227,228]
- active techniques (muscle contraction).

Many of the studies of sensory gating previously discussed demonstrated the principle that sensory gating is most effective when the gating stimulus is applied in the vicinity of the test stimulus. If the gating stimulus is movement of a limb, gating is most effective when movement is of the test limb, but less effective during active or passive movement of other limbs. This implies that manual gating should be close to the area of damage (pain). However, the manipulation has to be carried out without inflicting further pain.

Table 12.1 Possible gating of pain from different musculoskeletal structures by manipulation

Source of pain	Possible manual gating
Muscle–tendon pain	Direct massage to muscle Rhythmic shortening and elongation by joint articulation Rhythmic voluntary contraction
Joint pain	Rhythmic, oscillatory joint articulation
Ligament pain	Rhythmic elongation and shortening by joint articulation

For example, in joint effusion and pain, manual gating can take the form of joint articulation within the pain-free range. For example, in lateral strain of the ankle, the joint can be articulated into cycles of flexion and extension. Manual gating of muscle pain may be achieved by direct massage of the muscle, gentle non-painful cycles of muscle shortening and elongation (by joint movement), and possibly rhythmic muscle contractions.

In muscle, specialized nociceptors convey information about sustained increases in intramuscular pressure (mechanical irritation), temperature, muscle ischaemia[200] and chemical excitation.[229] These receptors are less sensitive to changes in muscle length, such as those from muscle stretching, or to muscle contraction.[200,229] The common observation that muscle pain can be reduced by stretching or contraction is possibly related to the stimulation of muscle mechanoreceptors to the exclusion of nociceptors. Pain relief may occur when the muscle's mechanoreceptors gate the pain sensation conveyed by the nociceptors.[229]

It remains to be evaluated which techniques are more effective for different painful conditions. The possible influence of touch on higher centres and its effects on pain perception are discussed in Section 3.

REDUCING THE POTENTIAL FOR ADVERSE REACTIONS

Hyperalgesia (hypersensitivity) and its implications for manual techniques

Following injury, the site of damage as well as its surrounding area will become hypersensitive to mechanical stimuli. Two mechanisms account for this. Peripherally, there is a reduction in the threshold of pain-conveying receptors as a result of inflammatory byproducts (see Section 1). Centrally, there is a functional reorganization within the spinal cord,[230] with an increase in sensitivity of various neurons.[231] Similar to the situation in peripheral sensitization, this central sensitization results in neurons responding to lower-intensity events to which they were previously insensitive.

The sensitivity brought about by noxious events tends to spread in the spinal cord.[232–234] The higher the intensity of peripheral irritation the further the spread and strength of sensitization within the spinal centres.[231] This spread of excitation has also been shown to reduce the threshold of motorneurons,[92] and therefore affect muscle activity around the site of injury. (This mechanism probably plays a part in the protective muscle splinting that is often seen during acute injury.) There is also a difference in the spread of sensitization caused by pain arising from superficial and deep receptors: in comparison with skin, pain from deep structures such as muscle and joints seems to produce greater central sensitization.[231]

The neurological mechanism described above should be taken into consideration during manipulation. Direct, painful manipulation to and around the damaged area may increase spinal sensitization and hyperalgesia, resulting in an adverse painful response. The overall aim of treatment should be to 'starve' the system of noxious excitation and reduce the state of hypersensitivity. For that purpose, non-painful manipulation should be used in treating certain pain conditions.

Nociceptors do not adapt to, or fatigue after, noxious mechanical stimuli

There are several manual techniques in which causing pain is seen as a form of hyperirritation, resulting in inhibition of pain. However, during inflammation, it has been demonstrated that pain will last as long as the mechanical irritation is applied, and that this sensation does not decrease with time.[201] This means that pain will increase during the period of manipulation and (by central sensitization) potentially outlast it. The only pain relief that takes place in these techniques is when manipulation is over and the pressure is removed! It is very likely that these types of technique cause further tissue damage rather then inhibiting pain or supporting the repair processes. Direct deep manipulation of the damaged area does not inhibit pain and should be avoided. However, direct manipulation to the area of damage may be beneficial in pain reduction by its effects on fluid dynamics (as discussed in Section 1). In these circumstances, pain should be minimized. Inflicting pain in the hope that it will reduce pain should *not* be the aim of treatment.

13

Overview and summary of Section 2

Section 2 of this book examined the role that manual therapy has in rehabilitation and normalization of the motor system. The functional organization of the motor system was examined, particular emphasis being paid to proprioceptors and their influence on the motor system. Manual techniques were neurologically classified into groups of active, passive, dynamic and static.

These different modes of manipulation were examined with respect to their potential influences on motor processes such as neuromuscular plasticity. It was argued that motor changes can only take place with an active-mode manual technique; passive techniques have little or no influence on motor events. However, passive techniques can start off many treatments in which patients are unable to carry out the movement themselves, or can guide patients during new movement patterns. Dynamic modes also seem to be more important than static ones in stimulating the motor system. In essence, active–dynamic techniques seem to have prominence over other forms of manipulation at this level of organization. However, these techniques should be closely related to motor processes such as motor abilities, motor learning and transfer principles.

Another principle that emerges from this section is that reflexive-type treatment aiming to stimulate the lower motor system (spinal reflexes) is ineffective as a treatment modality. More important, and possibly the only treatment approach to have any longlasting effect is one which communicates with the patient and encourages movement that is cognitive and voli-tional. The view of the individual as a collection of reflexes must fall. Indeed, much research in the past that examined complex spinal pathways has largely failed to contribute to neurorehabili-tation, except by demonstrating that this avenue is not a feasible treatment approach.

In normalizing the motor system, the therapist should accept the person as a whole, with the patient taking an active part and understanding his or her role in the healing process.

Motor and muscle tone have been differenti-ated and the causes of abnormal tone have been discussed. Motor tone is initiated by a command from the motor system, whereas muscle tone is created by local mechanical changes in the muscle. In a fully relaxed person, there is motor silence, and the tension in the muscle is mechan-ical in origin. It has been argued that the muscular tension often felt in musculoskeletal injuries results from an increase in mechanical pressure rather than from sustained neurological tone. However, any mechanical change in the muscle in a reflection of its function. The cause of the abnormal muscle tone should be identified and addressed during treatment.

Neurological pain mechanisms, in particular the role of manually induced analgesia, have been examined. It has been proposed that some of the pain relief seen during and follow-ing manipulation may be related to sensory gating.

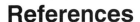

References

1. Butler D S 1991 Mobilisation of the nervous system. Churchill Livingstone, London
2. DeFeudis F V, DeFeudis P A F 1977 Elements of the behavioral code. Academic Press, London
3. Schmidt R A 1991 Motor learning and performance: from principles to practice. Human Kinetic Books, Champaign, II
4. Williams H G 1969 Neurological concepts and perceptual-motor behavior. In: Brown R C, Cratty B J (eds) New perspective of man in action. Prentice Hall, Englewood Cliffs, NJ
5. Goodwin G M, McCloskey D I, Matthews P B C 1972 The contribution of muscle afferents to kinaesthesia shown by vibration induced illusion of movement and the effects of paralysing joint afferents. Brain 95: 705–748
6. Henry F M, Rogers D E 1960 Increased response latency for complicated movements in a "memory drum" theory of neuromotor reaction. Research Quarterly 31: 448–458
7. Schmidt R A 1982 Motor learning and control: a behavioral emphasis. Human Kinetics, Champaign, IL
8. Dietz V 1992 Human neuronal control of automatic functional movements: interaction between central programs and afferent inputs. Physiological Reviews 72(1) :33–69
9. Grillner S, Zanggar P 1975 How detailed is the central pattern generator for locomotion. Brain Research 88: 367–371
10. McCloskey D I, Gandevia S C 1978 Role of inputs from skin, joints and muscles and of corollary discharges, in human discriminatory tasks. In: Gordon G (ed) Active touch. Pergamon Press Oxford, p 177–188
11. von-Holst E 1954 Relations between the central nervous system and the peripheral organs. British Journal of Animal Behaviour 2: 89–94
12. Laszlo J I, Bairstow P J 1971 Accuracy of movement, peripheral feedback and efferent copy. Journal of Motor Behaviour 3: 241–252
13. Dickson J 1974 Proprioceptive control of human movement. Lepus Books, London
14. Smith J L 1969 Kinesthesis: a model for movement feedback. In: Brown R C, Cratty B J (eds) New perspective of man in action. Prentice Hall, Englewood Cliffs, NJ

15. Gardner E P 1987 Somatosensory cortical mechanisms of feature detection in tactile and kinesthetic discrimination. Canadian Journal of Physiology and Pharmacology 66: 439–454
16. Matthews P B C 1988 Proprioceptors and their contribution to somatosensory mapping: complex messages require complex processing. Canadian Journal of Physiology and Pharmacology 66: 430–438
17. Wall P D 1960 Cord cells responding to touch, damage, and temperature of skin. Journal of Neurophysiology 23: 197–210
18. Wall P D 1975 The somatosensory system. In: Gazzaniga M S, Blackmore C (eds) Handbook of psychobiology. Academic Press, London
19. Sinclair D C 1955 Cutaneous sensation and the doctrine of specific energy. Brain 78: 584–614
20. Bennett D J, Gorassini M, Prochazka A 1994 Catching a ball: contribution of intrinsic muscle stiffness, reflexes, and higher order responses. Canadian Journal of Physiology and Pharmacology 72(2): 525–534
21. Roland P E 1978 Sensory feedback to the cerebral cortex during voluntary movement in man. Behavioral and Brain Sciences 1: 129–171
22. Lemon R N, Porter R 1978 Short-latency peripheral afferent inputs to pyramidal and other neurones in the precentral cortex of conscious monkeys. In: Gordon G (ed) Active touch. Pergamon Press, Oxford, p 91–103
23. Bobath B 1979 The application of physiological principles to stroke rehabilitation. The Practitioner 223: 793–794
24. Rothwell J C, Traub M M, Day B L, Obeso J A, Thomas P K, Marsden C D 1982 Manual performance in a de-afferented man. Brain 105: 515–542
25. Jones L A 1988 Motor illusions: what do they reveal about proprioception. Physiological Bulletin 103(1): 72–86
26. Vallbo A B, Hagbarth K-E, Torebjork H E, Wallin B G 1979 Somatosensory, proprioceptive and sympathetic activity in human peripheral nerve. Physiological Reviews 59(4): 919–957
27. Houk J C 1978 Participation of reflex mechanisms and reaction time processes in the compensatory adjustments to mechanical disturbances. Progress in Clinical Neurophysiology 4: 193–215
28. Gielen C C A M, Ramaekers L, van Zuylen E J 1988 Long latency stretch reflexes as co-ordinated functional responses in man. Journal of Physiology 407: 275–292
29. O'Sullivan M C, Eyre J A, Miller S 1991 Radiation of the phasic stretch reflex in biceps brachii to muscles of the arm in man and its restriction during development. Journal of Physiology 439: 529–543
30. Strick P L 1978 Cerebellar involvement in volitional muscle responses to load changes. Progress in Clinical Neurophysiology 4: 85–93
31. Matthews P B C 1991 The human stretch reflex and motor cortex. Trends in Neuro Science 14(3): 87–91
32. Rack P M H, Ross H F, Brown T I H 1978 Reflex responses during sinusoidal movement of human limbs. Progress in Clinical Neurophysiology 4: 216–228
33. Nashner L M, Grimm R J 1978 Analysis of multiloop dyscontrols in standing cerebellar patients. Progress in Clinical Neurophysiology 4: 300–319
34. Matthews P B C 1986 Observation on the automatic compensation of reflex gain on varying the pre-existing level of motor discharge in man. Journal of Physiology 374: 73–90
35. Bizzi E, Dev P, Morasso P, Polit A 1978 Role of neck proprioceptors during visually triggered head movements. Progress in Clinical Neurophysiology 4: 141–152
36. Held R 1968 Plasticity in sensorimotor coordination. In: Freedman S J (ed) The neuropsychology of spatially oriented behavior. Dorsey Press, Homewood, IL
37. Rock I, Harris C S 1967 Vision and touch. Scientific American 216: 96–107
38. Lee D N, Aronson E 1974 Visual proprioceptive control of standing in human infants. Perception and Psychophysics 15: 527–532
39. Fitzpatrick R, Burke D, Gandevia S C 1994 Task-dependent reflex responses and movement illusions evoked by galvanic vestibular stimulation in standing humans. Journal of Physiology 478(2): 363–372
40. Chernikoff R, Taylor F V 1952 Reaction time to kinesthetic stimulation resulting from sudden arm displacement. Journal of Experimental Psychology 43: 1–8
41. Desmedt J E, Godaux E 1978 Ballistic skilled movements: load compensation and patterning of the motor commands. Progress in Clinical Neurophysiology 4: 21–55
42. Cockerill I M 1972 The development of ballistic skill movements. In: Whiting H T A (ed) Readings in sports psychology. Henry Kimpton, London
43. Lashley K S 1917 The accuracy of movement in the absence of excitation from the moving organ. American Journal of Physiology 43: 169–194
44. Taub E 1976 Movement in nonhuman primates deprived of somatosensory feedback. Exercise and Sports Science Reviews 4: 335–374
45. Taub E, Berman A J 1968 Movement and learning in the absence of sensory feedback. In: The neurophysiology of spatially orientated behavior. Dorsey Press, Homewood, IL
46. Laszlo J I 1967 Training of fast tapping with reduction of kinaesthetic, tactile, visual and auditory sensations. Quarterly Journal of Experimental Psychology 19: 344–349
47. Von Euler C 1985 Central pattern generation during breathing. In: The motor system in neurobiology. Biomedical Press, Oxford
48. Rushton D N, Rothwell J C, Craggs M D 1981 Gating of somatosensory evoked potentials during different kinds of movement in man. Brain 104: 465–491
49. Granit R 1955 Receptors and sensory perception. Yale University Press, London
50. Wyke B D 1985 Articular neurology and manipulative therapy. In: Glasgow E F, Twomey L T, Scull E R, Kleynhans A M, Idczek R M (eds) Aspects of manipulative therapy. Churchill Livingstone, Edinburgh, ch 11, p 72–77
51. Jami L 1992 Golgi tendon organs in mammalian skeletal muscle: functional properties and central actions. Physiological Reviews 73(3): 623–666
52. Matthews P B C 1981 Muscle spindles: their messages and their fusimotor supply. In: Brookhart J M, Mountcastle V B, Brooks V B, Geiger S R (eds) Handbook of physiology, Section 1: The nervous

system, Volume 2: Motor control. American Physiological Society, Bethesda, M, ch 6

53. Carpenter R S H 1990 Neurophysiology. Edward Arnold, London

54. Vallbo A B 1968 Activity from skin mechanoreceptors recorded percutaneously in awake human subjects. Experimental Neurology 21: 270–289

55. Vallbo A B 1971 The muscle spindle response at the onset of isometric voluntary contractions in man. Time difference between fusimotor and skeletomotor effects. Journal of Physiology 318: 405–431

56. Burke D, Hagbarth K-E, Lofstedt L 1977 Muscle spindle activity in man during shortening and lengthening contractions. Journal of Physiology 277: 131–142

57. Burke D, Hagbarth K E, Lofstedt L 1978 Muscle spindle activity during shortening and lengthening contractions. Journal of Physiology 277: 131–142

58. Matthews P B C 1964 Muscle spindles and their motor control. Physiological Review 44: 219–288

59. Vallbo A B 1973 Afferent discharge from human muscle spindle in non-contracting muscles. Steady state impulse frequency as a function of joint angle. Acta Physiologica Scandinavica 90: 303–318

60. Millar J 1973 Joint afferent fibres responding to muscle stretch, vibration and contraction. Brain Research 63: 380 383

61. Berthoz A, Metral S 1970 Behaviour of a muscular group subjected to a sinusoidal and trapezoid variation of force. Journal of Applied Physiology 29(3): 378–383

62. Johansson H, Sjolander P, Sojka P 1991 Receptors in the knee and their role in the biomechanics of the joint. Critical Reviews in Biomedical Engineering 18(5): 341–368

63. Jenkins D H R 1985 Ligament injuries and their treatment. Chapman & Hall Medical, London

64. Ramcharan J E, Wyke B 1972 Articular reflexes at the knee joint: an electromyographic study. American Journal of Physiology 223(6): 1276–1280

65. Lee J, Ring P A 1954 The effect of local anaesthesia on the appreciation of passive movement in the great toe of man. Proceedings of the Physiological Society, p 56–57

66. Schaible H-G, Grubb B D 1993 Afferents and spinal mechanisms of joint pain. Pain 55: 5–54

67. Krauspe R, Schmidt M, Schaible H-G 1992 Sensory innervation of the anterior cruciate ligament. Journal of Bone and Joint Surgery (A) 74(3): 390–397

68. Wyke B 1967 The neurology of joints. Annals of the Royal College of Surgeons of England 42: 25–50

69. Coggeshall R E, Hong K A H P, Langford L A, Schaible H-G, Schmidt R F 1983 Discharge characteristics of fine medial articular afferents at rest and during passive movement of the inflamed knee joints. Brain Research 272: 185–188

70. Schaible H-G, Grubb B D 1993 Afferents and spinal mechanisms of joint pain. Pain 55: 5–54

71. Nielsen J, Pierrot-Deseilligny E 1991 Patterns of cutaneous inhibition of the propriospinal-like excitation to human upper limb motorneurons. Journal of Physiology 434: 169–182

72. Gandevia S C, McCloskey D I, Burke D 1992 Kinaesthetic signals and muscle contraction. Trends in Neuro Science 15(2): 64–65

73. Vallbo A B, Johansson R S 1978 The tactile sensory innnervation of the glabrous skin of the human hand. In: Gordon G (ed) Active touch. Pergamon Press, Oxford, p 29–54

74. Lloyd A J, Caldwell L S 1965 Accuracy of active and passive positioning of the leg on the basis of kinesthetic cues. Journal of Comparative and Physiological Psychology 60(1): 102–106

75. Paillard J, Brouchon M 1968 Active and passive movements in the calibration of position sense. In: Freedman S J (ed) The neuropsychology of spatially oriented behavior. Dorsey Press, Homewood, IL, p 37–55

76. Nauta W J H, Karten H J 1970 A general profile of the vertebrate brain with sidelights on the ancestry of cerebral cortex. In: Schmitt F O (ed) The neurosciences. Rockefeller University Press, New York, p 7–26

77. Forssberg H, Grillner S, Rossignol S 1975 Phase dependent reflex reversal during walking in chronic spinal cat. Brain Research 85: 103–107

78. Guyton A C 1981 Basic human physiology. W B Saunders, London

79. Phillips C G 1978 Significance of the monosynaptic cortical projection to spinal motorneurones in primates. Progress in Clinical Neurophysiology 4: 21–55

80. Luscher H-R, Clamann H P 1992 Relation between structure and function in information transfer in spinal monosynaptic reflex. Physiological Reviews 72(1): 71–99

81. Noback C R, Demarest R J 1981 The human nervous system: basic principles of neurobiology, 3rd edn. McGraw-Hill, New York

82. Cody F W J, Plant T 1989 Vibration evoked reciprocal inhibition between human wrist muscles. Brain Research 78: 613 623

83. Mathews P B C 1966 The reflex excitation of of the soleus muscle of decerebrated cat caused by vibration applied to its tendon. Journal of Physiology 184: 450–472

84. Eklund G, Steen M 1969 Muscle vibration therapy in children with cerebral palsy. Scandinavian Journal of Rehabilitation and Medicine 1: 35–37

85. Burke D, Andrews C J, Gillies J D 1971 The reflex response to sinusoidal stretching in spastic man. Brain 94: 455–470

86. Hagbarth K E, Eklund G 1969 The muscle vibrator: a useful tool in neurological therapeutic work. Scandinavian Journal of Rehabilitation and Medicine 1: 26–34

87. Hagbarth K E 1973 The effect of muscle vibration in normal man and in patients with motor disorders. New Developments in Electromyography and Clinical Neurophysiology 3: 428–443

88. Issacs E R, Szumski A J, Suter C 1968 Central and peripheral influences on the H-reflex in normal man. Neurology 18: 907–914

89. Burke D, Dickson H G, Skuse N F 1991 Task dependent changes in the responses to low-threshold cutaneous afferent volleys in the human lower limb. Journal of Physiology 432: 445–458

90. Sojka P, Sjolander P, Johansson H, Djupsjobacka M 1991 Influence from stretch sensitive receptors in the collateral ligaments of the knee joint on the gamma muscle spindle system of flexor and extensor muscles. Neuroscience Research 11: 55 62

91. Freeman M A R, Wyke B 1967 Articular reflexes at the ankle joint: an electromyographic study of normal and abnormal influences on ankle joint mechanoreceptors upon reflex activity in the leg muscles. British Journal of Surgery 54(12): 990–1000

92. He X, Proske U, Schaible H-G, Shmidt R F 1988 Acute inflammation of the knee joint in the cat alters responses of flexor motorneurons to leg movements. Journal of Neurophysiology 59: 326–339

93. Johansson H, Lorentzon R, Sjolander P, Sjoka P 1990 The anterior cruciate ligament. A sensor acting on the gamma muscle-spindle systems of muscles around the knee joint. Neuro-Orthopedics 9: 1–23

94. Grigg P, Harrigan E P, Fogearty K E 1978 Segemental reflexes mediated by joint afferent neurons in cat knee. Journal of Neurophysiology 41(1): 9–14

95. Baxendale R H, Farrell W R 1981 The effect of knee joint afferent discharge on transmission in flexion reflex pathways in decerebrate cats. Journal of Physiology 315: 231–242

96. Evarts E V 1980 Brain mechanisms in voluntary movement. In: Mcfadden D (ed) Neural mechanisms in behavior. Springer-Verlag, New York

97. Capaday C, Stein R B 1986 Difference in the amplitude of the human soleus H-reflex during walking and running. Journal of Physiology 392: 513–522

98. Lundberg A, Malmgren K, Schomberg E D 1978 Role of joint afferents in motor control exemplified by effects on reflex pathway from 1b afferents. Journal of Physiology 284: 327–343

99. Kukulka C G, Beckman S M, Holte J B, Hoppenworth P K 1986 Effects of intermittent tendon pressure on alpha motorneuron exitability. Physical Therapy 66(7): 1091–1094

100. Leone J A, Kukulka C G 1988 Effects of tendon pressure on alpha motorneuron excitability in patients with strokes. Physical Therapy 68(4): 475–480

101. Cody F W J, MacDermott N, Ferguson I T 1987 Stretch and vibration reflexes of wrist flexor muscles in spasticity. Brain 110: 433–450

102. Belanger A Y, Morin S, Pepin P, Tremblay M-H, Vacho J 1989 Manual muscle tapping decreases soleus H-reflex amplitude in control subjects. Physiotherapy Canada 41(4): 192–196

103. Sullivan S J, Williams L R T, Seaborne D E, Morelli M 1991 Effects of massage on alpha neuron excitability. Physical Therapy 71(8): 555–560

104. Goldberg J 1992 The effect of two intensities of massage on H-reflex amplitude. Physical Therapy 72(6): 449–457

105. Goldberg J, Seaborne D E, Sullivan S J, Leduc B E 1994 The effect of therapeutic massage on H-reflex amplitude in persons with a spinal cord injury. Physical Therapy 74(8): 728–737

106. Guissard N, Duchateau J, Hainaut K 1988 Muscle stretching and motorneuron excitability. European Journal of Applied Physiology 58: 47–52

107. Sullivan S J, Seguin S, Seaborne D, Goldberg J 1993 Reduction of H-reflex amplitude during the application of effleurage to the triceps surae in neurologically healthy subjects. Physiotherapy Theory and Practice 9: 25–31

108. Darton K, Lippold O C J, Shahani M, Shahani U 1985 Long latency spinal reflexes in humans. Journal of Neurophysiology 53:(6): 1604–1618

109. Humphrey D R, Reed D J 1983 Separate cortical systems for control of joint movement and joint stiffness: reciprocal activation and coactivation of antagonist muscles. Advances in Neurology 39: 347–372

110. Hayes K C, Sullivan J 1976 Tonic neck reflex influence on tendon and Hoffmann reflexes in man. Electromyography and Clinical Neurophysiology 16: 251–261

111. Badke M B, DiFabio R P 1984 Facilitation: new theoretical perspective and clinical approach. In: Basmajian J V, Wolf S L (eds) Therapeutic exercise. Williams & Wilkins, London p 77–91

112. Magill R A 1985 Motor learning concepts and applications. William C Brown, Iowa

113. Fitts P M, Posner M I 1967 Human performance. Brooks/Cole California

114. Wrisberg C A, Shea C H 1978 Shifts in attention demands and motor program utilization during motor learning. Journal of Motor Behavior 10: 149–158

115. Rose S 1992 The making of memory: from molecules to mind. Bantam Books, London

116. Kidd G, Lawes N, Musa I 1992 Understanding neuromuscular plasticity: a basis for clinical rehabilitation. Edward Arnold, London

117. Pascual-Leone A, Cohen L G, Hallet M 1992 Cortical map plasticity in humans. Trends in Neuro Science 15(1): 13–14

118. Merzenich M M 1984 Functional maps of skin sensations. In: Brown C C (ed) The many faces of touch. Johnson & Johnson Baby Products Company Pediatric Round Table Series, 10, p 15–22

119. Wolpaw J R 1985 Adaptive plasticity in the spinal stretch reflex: an accessible substrate of memory? Cellular and Molecular Neurobiology 5(1/2): 147–165

120. Wolpaw J R, Lee C L 1989 Memory traces in primate spinal cord produced by operant conditioning of H-reflex. Journal of Neurobiology 61(3): 563–573

121. Wolpaw J R, Carp J S, Lam Lee C 1989 Memory traces in spinal cord produced by H-reflex conditioning: effects of post-tetanic potentiation. Neuroscience Letters 103: 113–119

122. Evatt M L, Wolf S L, Segal R L 1989 Modification of the human stretch reflex: preliminary studies. Neuroscience Letters 105: 350–355

123. Hodgson J A, Roland R R, de-Leon R, Dobkin B, Reggie Edgerton V 1994 Can the mammalian lumbar spinal cord learn a motor task? Medicine and Science in Sports and Exercise 26(12): 1491–1497

124. McComas A J 1994 Human neuromuscular adaptations that accompany changes in activity. Medicine and Science in Sports and Exercise 26(12): 1498–1509

125. Kahneman D 1973 Attention and effort. Prentice Hall, Englewood Cliffs, NJ

126. Adams J A 1966 Short-term memory for motor responses. Journal of Experimental Psychology 71(2): 314–318

127. Kottke F J et al 1978 The training of coordination. Archives of Physical and Medical Rehabilitation 59: 567–572

128. Wolpaw J R 1994 Acquisition and maintenance of the simplest motor skill: investigation of CNS mechanisms. Medicine and Science in Sports and Exercise 26(12): 1475–1479

129. Rose S P R, Hambley J, Haywood J 1976 Neurochemical approaches to developmental plasticity and learning. In: Rosenzweig M R, Bennett E Y L (eds) Neural mechanisms on learning and memory. MTI Press, Cambridge, MA

130. Morris S L, Sharpe M H 1993 PNF revisited. Physiotherapy Theory and Practice 9: 43–51

131. Holding D H 1965 Principles of training. Pergamon Press, London

132. Osgood C E 1949 The similarity paradox in human learning: a resolution. Psychology Review 56: 132–143

133. Fleishman E A 1966 Human abilities and the acquisition of skills. In: Bilodeau E A (ed) Acquisition of skill. Academic Press, New York

134. Fleishman E A 1964 The structure and measurement of physical fitness. Prentice Hall, Engelwood Cliffs, NJ

135. Alvares K M, Hulin C L 1972 Two explanations of temporal changes in ability–skill relationship: a literature review and theoretical analysis. Human Factors 14: 295–308

136. Slater-Hammel A T 1956 Performance of selected group of male college students on the Reynolds balance tests. Research Quarterly 27: 348–351.

137. Gross E A, Thompson H L 1957 Relationship of dynamic balance to speed and to ability in swimming. Research Quarterly 28: 342–346

138. Mumby H H 1953 Kinesthetic acuity and balance related to wrestling ability. Research Quarterly 24: 327–330

139. Sale D G 1988 Neural adaptation to resistance training. Medicine and Science in Sports and Exercise 20: 5

140. Beard D J, Dodd C A F, Trundle H R, Hamishi A, Simpson R W 1994 Proprioception enhancement for anterior cruciate ligament deficiency. Journal of Bone and Joint Surgery (B) 76: 654–659

141. Freeman M A R, Dean M R E, Hanham I W F 1965 The etiology and prevention of functional instability of the foot. Journal of Bone and Joint Surgery (B) 47(4): 678–685

142. Basmajian J V 1978 Muscles alive: their function revealed by electromyography. Williams & Wilkins, Baltimore

143. Markolf K L, Graff-Radford A, Amstutz H 1979 In vivo knee stability. A quantitive assessment using an instrumental clinical testing apparatus. Journal of Bone and Joint Surgery (A) 60: 664–674

144. Panjabi M M 1992 The stabilizing system of the spine. Part 1. Function, dysfunction, adaptation, and enhancement. Journal of Spinal Disorders 5(4): 383–389

145. Yamazaki Y, Ohkuwa T, Suzuki M 1994 Reciprocal activation and coactivation in antagonistic muscle during rapid goal-directed movement. Brain Research Bulletin 34(6): 587–593

146. Psek J A, Cafarelli E 1993 Behavior of coactive muscles during fatigue. Journal of Applied Physiology 74(1): 170–175

147. Feldenkrais M 1983 The elusive obvious. Aleff Publications, Tel-Aviv

148. Vorro J, Wilson F R, Dainis A 1978 Multivariate analysis of biomechanical profiles for the coracobrachialis and biceps brachii muscles in humans. Ergonomics 21: 407–418

149. Jacobson E 1932 Electrophysiology of mental activity. American Journal of Psychology 44: 676–694

150. Kelsey B 1961 Effects of mental practice and physical practice upon muscular endurance. Research Quarterly 32(99): 47–54

151. Rawlings E I, Rawlings I L, Chen C S, Yilk M D 1972 The facilitating effects of mental rehearsal in the acquisition of rotary pursuit tracking. Psychonomic Science 26: 71–73

152. Yue G, Cole K J 1992 Strength increases from the motor programme: comparison of training with maximal voluntary and imagined muscle contraction. Journal of Neurophysiology 67(5): 1114–1123

153. Dickinson J 1966 The training of mobile balancing under a minimal visual cue situation. Ergonomics 11: 169–175

154. Holding D H, Macrae A W 1964. Guidance, restriction and knowledge of results. Ergonomics 7: 289–295

155. Annett J 1959 Learning a pressure under conditions of immediate and delayed knowledge of results. Quarterly Journal of Experimental Psychology 11: 3–15

156. Gandevia S C, McCloskey D I 1976 Joint sense, muscle sense and their combination as position sense, measured at the distal interphalangeal joint of the middle finger. Journal of Physiology 260: 387–407

157. Ralston H J, Libet B 1953 The question of tonus in skeletal muscles. American Journal of Physical Medicine 32: 85–92

158. von-Wright J M 1957 A note on the role of guidance in learning. British Journal of Psychology 48: 133–137

159. Lincoln R S 1956 Learning and retaining a rate of movement with the aid of kinaesthetic and verbal cues. Journal of Experimental Psychology 51: 3

160. Cleghorn T E, Darcus H A 1952 The sensibility to passive movement of the human elbow joint. Quarterly Journal of Experimental Psychology 4: 66–77

161. Dalkiran J, Lederman E 1996 Unpublished observations

162. Cratty B J 1967 Movement behaviour and motor learning, 2nd ed, Henry Kimpton, London

163. Skinner H B et al 1984 Joint position sense in total knee arthroplasty. Journal of Orthopedic Research 1: 276–283

164. Hurley M V, Newham D J 1993 The influence of arthrogenous muscle inhibition on quadriceps rehabilitation of patients with early, unilateral osteoarthritic knees. British Journal of Rheumatology 32: 127–131

165. Barrack R L, Skinner H B, Cook S D, Haddad R S 1983 Effect of articular disease and total knee arthroplasty on knee joint-position sense. Journal of Neurophysiology 50(3): 684–687

166. Barrett D S, Cobb A G, Bentley G 1991 Joint proprioception in normal, osteoarthritic and replaced knee. Journal of Bone and Joint Surgery (B) 73(1): 53–56

167. Barrack R L, Skinner H B, Buckley S L 1989 Proprioception in the anterior cruciate deficient knee. American Journal of Sports Medicine 17(1): 1–6

168. Parkhurst T M, Burnett C N 1994 Injury and proprioception in the lower back. Journal of Orthopaedic and Sports Physical Therapy 19(5): 282–295

169. Glencross D, Thornton E 1981 Position sense following injury. Journal of Sports Medicine 21: 23–27

170. Isacsson G, Isberg A, Persson A 1988 Loss of directional orientation control of lower jaw movements in persons with internal derangement of the temporomandibular joint. Oral Surgery 66(1): 8–12

171. Thomas P A, Andriacchhi T P, Galante J O, Fermier R N 1982 Influence of total knee replacement design on walking and stair climbing. Journal of Bone and Joint Surgery (A) 64(9): 1328–1335

172. Stauffer R N, Chao E Y S, Gyory A N 1977 Biomechanical gait analysis of the diseased knee joint. Clinical Orthopedics 126: 246–255

173. Barrack R L 1991 Proprioception and function after anterior cruciate reconstruction. Journal of Bone and Joint Surgery (B) 73: 833–837

174. Ryan L 1994 Mechanical stability, muscle strength and proprioception in the functionally unstable ankle. Australian Journal of Physiotherapy 40: 41–47

175. Skinner H B, Wyatt M P, Hodgdon J A, Conard D W, Barrack R L 1986 Effect of fatigue on joint position sense of the knee. Journal of Orthopedic Research 4: 112–118

176. Marks R 1994 Effects of exercise-induced fatigue on position sense of the knee. Australian Physiotherapy 40(3): 175–181

177. Johansson H, Djupsjobacka M, Sjolander P 1993 Influence on the gamma-muscle spindle system from muscle afferents stimulated by KCl and lactic acid. Neuroscience Research 16(1): 49–57

178. Matsumoto D E, Baker J H 1987 Degeneration and alteration of axons and intrafusal muscle fibres in spindles following tenotomy. Experimental Neurology 97: 482–498

179. Vrbova M C I, Westbury D R 1977 The sensory reinnervation of hind limb muscles of the cat following denervation and de-efferentation. Neuroscience 2: 423–434

180. Maier A, Eldred E, Edgerton V R 1972 The effect on spindles of muscles atrophy and hypertrophy. Experimental Neurology 37: 100–123

181. Kennedy J C, Alexander I J, Hayes K C 1982 Nerve supply of the human knee and its functional importance. American Journal of Sports Medicine 10(6): 329–335

182. Jones D W, Jones D A, Newham D J 1987 Chronic knee effusion and aspiration: the effect on quadriceps inhibition. British Journal of Rheumatology 26: 370–374

183. Iles J F, Stokes M, Young A 1990 Reflex actions of knee joint afferents during contraction of the human quadriceps. Clinical Physiology 10: 489–500

184. Stokes M, Young A 1984 The contribution of reflex inhibition to arthrogenous muscle weakness. Clinical Science 67: 7–14

185. Spencer J D, Hayes K C Alexander I J 1984 Knee joint effusion and quadriceps reflex inhibition in man. Archives of Physical and Medical Rehabilitation 65: 171–177

186. Solomonow M, Baratta R, Zhou B H et al 1987 The synergistic action of the anterior cruciate ligament and thigh muscles in maintaining joint stability. American Journal of Sports Medicine 15(3): 207–213

187. Hurley M V, O'Flanagan S J, Newham D J 1991 Isokinetic and isometric muscle strength and inhibition after elbow arthroplasty. Journal of Orthopedic Rheumatology 4: 83–95

188. Alexander R, Bennet-Clerk H C 1977 Storage of elastic energy in muscles and other tissues. Nature 265: 114–117

189. Tangelder G J, Slaaf D W, Reneman R S 1984 Skeletal muscle microcirculation and changes in transmural perfusion pressure. Progress in Applied Microcirculation 5: 93–108

190. Baumann J U, Sutherland D H, Hangg A 1979 Intramuscular pressure during walking: an experimental study using the wick catheter technique. Clinical Orthopedics and Related Research 145: 292–299

191. Kirkebo A, Wisnes A 1982 Regional tissue fluid pressure in rat calf muscle during sustained contraction or stretch. Acta Physiologica Scandinavica 114: 551–556

192. Sejersted O M et al 1984 Intramuscular fluid pressure during isometric contraction of human skeletal muscle. Journal of Applied Physiology 56(2): 287–295

193. Petrofsky J S, Hendershot D M 1984 The interrelationship between bloodpressure, intramuscular pressure, and isometric endurance in fast and slow twitch muscle in the cat. European Journal of Applied Physiology 53: 106–111

194. Hill A V 1948 The pressure developed in muscle during contraction. Journal of Physiology 107: 518–526

195. Basmajian J V 1957 New views on muscular tone and relaxation. Canadian Medical Association Journal 77: 203–205

196. Clemmesen S 1951 Some studies of muscle tone. Proceedings of the Royal Society of Medicine 44: 637–646

197. Gardner A M N, Fox R H, Lawrence C, Bunker T D, Ling R S M, MacEachern A G 1990 Reduction of post-traumatic swelling and compartment pressure by impulse compression of the foot. Journal of Bone and Joint Surgery (B) 72: 810–815

198. Lennox C M E 1993 Muscle injuries. In: McLatchie G R, Lennox C M E (eds) Soft tissues: trauma and sports injuries. Butterworth Heinemann, London, p 83–103

199. McMahon S, Koltzenburg M 1990 Novel classes of nociceptors: beyond Sherrington. Trends in Neuro Science 13(6): 199–201

200. Casey K L 1978 Neural mechanisms of pain. In: Carterette E C, Friedman M P (eds) Handbook of perception: feeling and hurting. Academic Press, London, ch 6, p 183–219

201. Meyer R A, Campbell J A, Raja S 1994 Peripheral neural mechanisms of nociception. In: Wall P D, Melzack R (eds) Textbook of pain, 3rd edn. Churchill Livingstone, London, p 13–42

202. Paalasmaa P, Kemppainen P, Pertovaara A 1991 Modulation of skin sensitivity by dynamic and isometric exercise in man. Applied Physiology 62: 279–283

203. Milne R J, Aniss A M, Kay N E, Gandevia S C 1988 Reduction in perceived intensity of cutaneous stimuli during movement: a quantitative study. Experimental Brain Research 70: 569–576

204. Dyhre-Poulsen P 1978 Perception of tactile stimuli before ballistic and during tracking movements. In: Gordon G (ed) Active touch. Pergamon Press, Oxford, p 171–176

205. Craig J C 1978 Vibrotactile pattern recognition and masking. In: Gordon G (ed) Active touch. Pergamon Press, Oxford, p 229–242

206. Ghez C, Pisa M 1972 Inhibition of afferent transmission in cuneate nucleus during voluntary movement in the cat. Brain Research 40: 145–151

207. Chapman C E, Bushnell M C, Miron D, Duncan G H, Lund J P 1987 Sensory perception during movement in man. Experimental Brain Research 68: 516–524

208. Angel R W, Weinrich M, Siegler D 1985 Gating of somatosensory perception following movement. Experimental Neurology 90: 395–400

209. Hochreiter N W, Jewell M J, Barber L, Browne P 1983 Effects of vibration on tactile sensitivity. Physical Therapy 63(6): 934–937

210. Feine J S, Chapman C E, Lund J P, Duncan G H, Bushnell M C 1990 The perception of painful and nonpainful stimuli during voluntary motor activity in man. Somatosensory and Motor Research 7(2): 113–124

211. Wall P D, Cronly-Dillon J R 1960 Pain, itch and vibration. American Medical Archives of Neurology 2: 365–375

212. Lundeberg T, Ottoson D, Hakansson S, Meyerson B A 1983 Vibratory stimulation for the control of intractable chronic orofacial pain. Advances in Pain Research and Therapy 5: 555–561

213. Ottoson D, Ekblom A, Hansson P 1981 Vibratory stimulation for the relief of pain of dental origin. Pain 10: 37–45

214. Lundeberg T, Nordemar R, Ottoson D 1984 Pain alleviation by vibratory stimulation. Pain 20: 25–44

215. Lundeberg T 1984 Long-term results of vibratory stimulation as a pain relieving measure for chronic pain. Pain 20: 13–23

216. Melzack R 1981 Myofascial trigger points: relation to acupuncture and mechanisms of pain. Archives of Physical and Medical Rehabilitation 62: 114–117

217. Melzack R, Wall P D 1965 Pain mechanisms: a new theory. Science 150: 971–979

218. Wall P D 1967 The laminar organization of dorsal horn and effects of descending impulses. Journal of Physiology 188: 403–423

219. Richardson D E 1976 Brain stimulation for pain control. IEEE Transactions on Biomedical Engineering 23(4): 304–306

220. Andersen P, Eccles J C, Sears T A 1964 Cortically evoked depolarization of primary afferents fibres in the spinal cord. Journal of Neurophysiology 27: 63–77

221. Reynolds D G 1969 Surgery in the rat during electrical analgesia induced by focal brain stimulation. Science 164: 444–445

222. Coquery J-M 1978 Role of active movement in control of afferent input from skin in cat and man. In: Gordon G (ed) Active touch. Pergamon Press, Oxford, p 161–170

223. Russell W R, Spalding J M K 1950 Treatment of painful amputation stumps. British Medical Journal 8: 68–73

224. Hansson P, Ekblom A 1981 Acute pain relieved by vibratory stimulus. British Dental Journal 6: 213

225. Hannington-Kiff J G 1981 Pain. Update Publications, London

226. Clelland J, Savinar E, Shepard K F 1987 The role of the physical therapist in chronic pain management. In: Burrows G P, Elton D, Stanley G V (eds) Handbook of chronic pain management. Elsevier, London, p 243–258

227. Zusman M, Edwards B C, Donaghy A 1989 Investigation of a proposed mechanism for the pain relief of spinal pain with passive joint movement. Journal of Manual Medicine 4: 58–61

228. Zusman M 1988 Prolonged relief from articular soft tissue pain with passive joint movement. Manual Medicine 3: 100–102

229. Mense S, Schmidt R F 1974 Activation of group IV afferent units from muscle by algesic agents. Brain Research 72: 305–310

230. Woolf C J 1994 The dorsal horn: state-dependent sensory processing and the generation of pain. In: Wall P D, Melzack R (eds) Textbook of pain, 3rd edn. Churchill Livingstone, London, p 101–112

231. Dubner R, Basbaum A I 1994 Spinal dorsal horn plasticity following tissue or nerve injury. In: Wall P D, Melzack R (eds) Textbook of pain, 3rd edn. Churchill Livingstone, London, p 225–242

232. Dunbar R, Ruda M A 1992 Activity-dependent neuronal plasticity following tissue injury and inflammation. Trends in Neuro Science 15(3): 96–103

233. Hylden J L K, Nahin R L, Traub R J, Dbner R 1989 Expension of receptive fields of spinal lamina I projection neurons in rat with unilateral adjuvant-induced inflammation: the contribution of dorsal horn mechanisms. Pain 37: 229–243

234. Cook A J, Woolf C J, Wall P D, MacMahon S 1987 Dynamic receptive field plasticity in rat spinal dorsal horn following C-primary afferent input. Nature 325: 151–153

235. Gray's Anatomy 1980 Williams P L, Warwick R (eds) Churchill Livingstone, London, p 859

Psychological and psychophysiological processes in manual therapy

14

Introduction to Section 3

Although manipulation starts at a local anatomical site, its remote influence on the human experience can be as far as the infinite expansion of the psyche. Manipulation is not limited by anatomical boundaries but involves the abstract world of the imagination, emotions, thoughts and full-life experience of the individual. Blankenburg[1] describes the body as 'the centre of orientation in our perception of our environment, focus of subjective experience, field of reference for subjective feelings, organ of expression and articulatory node between the self and the environment'. When we touch the patient, we touch the whole of this experience. Manipulation is not just a peripheral event involving a patch of skin, a joint here and there, a group of muscles, but a potential catalyst for remote psychological responses.

Several psychological changes can often be observed following a manual treatment:

- changes in perception of body image
- mood changes
- behavioural changes.

The influence of touch may not end there: most, if not all, emotions are associated with patterned somatic (psychosomatic or psychophysiological) responses, which may be quite varied:

- general changes in muscle tone
- altered autonomic and visceral activity
- increased pain tolerance
- the facilitation of healing processes
- the facilitation of self-regulation.

These effects are 'whole-person' responses, beyond the direct effects of manipulation on local tissue physiology and repair (as described in Section 1). This section will examine these whole-person processes.

Many of the responses described above can be viewed as a sequence, which starts in the body as a sensation from the area being manipulated. This sensation can bring about a psychological experience that will lead to a physiological and somatic change (Fig. 14.1). Although this sequence is a continuum, it can be artificially divided into two parts:

1. The *somatopsyche* sequence: This part of the sequence starts with the body as the source of sensory experience and its psychological influences and is discussed in Chapter 15.

2. The *psychosomatic* sequence: In this part of the sequence, the psychological responses to touch are transmitted and expressed in the body and is discussed in Chapter 16.

In Chapter 15, the somatopsyche sequence looks at how different forms of touch and movement are perceived and interpreted by the receiver, how touching the body 'touches the psyche.' It starts by considering the skin as a sensor, as well as other proprioceptive pathways where these sensations arise. It then moves on to touch as a form of communication, and its nurturing influences as well as the relationships between touch and emotion, body-self, body image, well-being, and health and touch as a therapeutic process. This is followed by the psychosomatic pathway in Chapter 16, examining how emotion is transmitted to the rest of the body as a somatic response. It looks in

Touch and manipulation

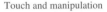

Proprioception

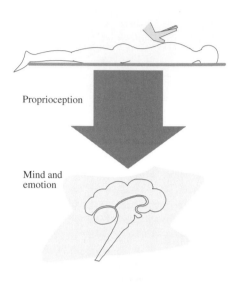

Mind and emotion

Somatization

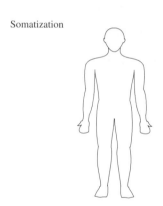

Figure 14.1 The proprioceptive-psychosomatic pathway (or somatic-psychosomatic pathway).

particular at three physiological pathways by which this transmission occurs.

15

The somatopsyche sequence

MANIPULATION AS SENSORY EXPERIENCE

All experiences depend on our sensory faculties: one cannot experience an event without sensory perception. Even 'internal' experiences such as dreaming or imagining are rooted in previous sensory experiences. Manipulation is also a sensory event. During manipulation, the individual is touched, stretched or articulated by the therapist, stimulating various receptors in the musculoskeletal system and skin.

The main receptors to be stimulated by manipulation are proprioceptors, which are found in muscles, tendons, joint capsules, ligaments and skin. They convey information about the mechanical state of the body, such as the velocity of movement, position of the joints, force of muscle contraction, length of muscle or mechanical events on the skin, for example deformation of the skin by massage or stretching. The anatomy and physiology of the different receptors have been extensively discussed in Section 2.

Although proprioceptors work in concert rather than singly, in order to understand the effect of manipulation on psychological processes, proprioception can be divided into two anatomical levels:

1. Superficial proprioception: sensations arising from the level of the skin, i.e. the body's envelope.

2. Deep proprioception: sensations arising from receptors in the muscles and joints complexes, i.e. the body's interior.

Various manual techniques will stimulate different levels of proprioception. Soft-tissue and massage techniques will stimulate the more superficial level of proprioception, whereas manual techniques using joint movement, stretching or deep kneading will stimulate the deep level of proprioception (Table 15.1). Manipulation of each of these levels will evoke sensory experiences that may hold different meanings for the patient. The emotions associated with stimulation of the superficial skin layer will be somewhat different from those of such stimulation as movement and stretching in the deeper proprioceptive level. These differences and similarities between the levels will be explored in the first part of this Section.

DEVELOPMENT OF PROPRIOCEPTION IN EARLY LIFE

The sense of touch is the first to become functional in embryonic life and is followed by proprioception and vestibular reflexes. Early sensory stimulation of the fetus is provided by the warmth and rhythmic activity that encompasses the womb: the heart beat, respiratory rhythms, peristalsis and movement of the body in daily activities.[2] All of these movements 'manipulate' the fetus, providing tactile stimulation of the skin. By the seventh week of intrauterine life the skin begins to provide sensation, appearing first in the lips and ending with the hands and feet. The top and back of the head remain insensitive to touch until birth.[3] There is some physiological evidence that, in infants, the maturation (myelination) of sensory afferents from the skin is the first to be completed, followed by that of vestibular, auditory and visual pathways.[4]

The rhythmic activity enfolding the fetus also stimulates deep proprioception by imposing passive movements on the fetus's limbs and trunk. Further deep proprioception arises from the fetus's own movements, which are performed against the resistance of the womb. Vestibular and proprioceptive responses can be observed in the human embryo about 2 weeks after the tactile skin responses (i.e. at about 9.5 weeks).[3]

Following birth, there is a continuation of both forms of proprioceptive stimulation by the infant's own movement and by extensive handling from the parent.

TOUCH AND MOVEMENT AS A STIMULUS FOR DEVELOPMENT AND SELF-REGULATION

Touch and movement have a nurturing effect on psychological and physical development. The nurturing effects of touch can be seen in premature infants, childhood and adulthood. In the young, tactile contact has been equated with feeding in its level of importance for normal development.[5,6] There are several anecdotal reports of the effects of manipulation on an individual's well-being and development. In one such report, there is a description of the effect of manual therapy on a young disabled child (part of the Rosemary project by the British School of Osteopathy).[7] When the child was referred for treatment, he suffered a host of problems: he was almost constantly crying, he had no verbal communication or eye contact, there was some uncertainty as to whether he was blind or deaf, he was unable to walk, had asthma, a constant runny nose and constant constipation, and he would not allow anyone to touch his head or neck. The manual treatment consisted of

Table 15.1 Examples of some common manual techniques and the level of proprioception they affect

Level of proprioception	Manual technique
Superficial proprioception	Soft tissue Massage (light) Effleurage Static holding techniques: cranial and functional
Deep proprioception	All techniques involving joint movement All active techniques where there is muscle contraction Stretching: longitudinal or cross-fibre Deep soft-tissue and massage techniques

massage, soft-tissue techniques, articulation and holding techniques (cranial and functional). In what seems to be a response to treatment, the child's crying reduced, his asthma attacks lessened, his digestion improved, non-verbal communication developed and he began to stand, walk and eventually climb stairs. He had fewer infections and began to interact and make friends.

Physical and tactile contacts are also important for reducing arousal and promoting self-regulation (Fig. 15.1).[8,9] The reduction in arousal by physical contact cannot be easily replaced by other means of comforting. This was partly demonstrated when an infant monkey was given the choice of feeding from one of two surrogate mothers, one made of wire and the other of cloth. The young monkey invariably preferred the cloth surrogate mother even when food was administered by the wire mother.[10,11] In times of distress, the monkey would run to its cloth mother and rub its body against 'hers', this intimate contact tending to calm the monkey. It would then turn to look at the objects that had previously terrified it, or explore them without the slightest sign of alarm. It was also found that the infant monkey preferred the unheated, cooler cloth mother in comparison to the floor of their cage which was warmed. These studies demonstrate that the attachment behaviour of the infant monkey to the surrogate mother was not related to satisfying hunger or physical warmth but to an instinctive need for contact comfort and tactile stimulation of a particular type. Similar behaviour can be observed in human infants.

When frightened, they tend to run and cling to their parent. Furthermore, like the infant monkey, human infants will replace or complement contact comfort by attachment behaviour towards a particular soft toy or a blanket.

TOUCH AND MOVEMENT DEPRIVATION

The importance of touch for normal development is more apparent when an animal or an individual is deprived of touch. There are several studies demonstrating this effect. However, it should be noted that the study of physical deprivation is highly complex. It is very difficult to study touch in isolation from other sources of deprivation, such as those of social and emotional contact.

During early life

Touch and kinesthetic deprivation can be seen in premature babies who are placed in an incubator and are deprived of the normal stimulation a full-term baby would normally receive in the womb. It is therefore possible to demonstrate how the introduction of touch can affect the infant's development and well-being. For example, gentle stroking of the infant combined with passive limb movements, has been shown to facilitate weight gain.[12,13] These infants were more active and alert and showed gains in behavioural development compared with the control group (neonates who did not receive tactile stimulation).[14] The overall hospital stay of the

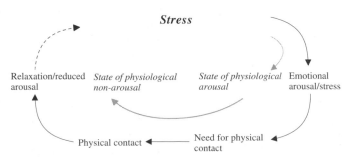

Figure 15.1   Physical contact as a means of reducing arousal.

study group was also 6 days shorter than that of the control group. In another study, static touch was provided to mechanically ventilated preterm infants by placing the hands on the infant's head and abdomen. The group of infants receiving touch required less oxygen and had a significantly higher red blood cell count.[15] Touch was also shown to reduce the number of apnoeic episodes (cessation of breathing) in very young premature infants.[16]

In children

Touch deprivation in early childhood also seems to retard normal development.[17–19] Such children show low intellectual and stunted physical development (for example, being underweight), are more prone to recurrent infection, ailments and accidents, and have a higher than normal mortality rate.[20,21] These effects of deprivation occur in children who are fed regularly and kept in high levels of hygiene. In contrast, babies with the longest mother contact have higher scores on intelligence;[22] they tend to cry less, smile more and perform better on developmental testing.[23] It has also been suggested that touch deprivation in childhood may play a part in mental illness later in life.[20]

Movement stimulation is also very important for the developing child. A child not stimulated by movement and deprived of touch may become still and resigned, and fail to cry appropriately. Sometimes the child may substitute the lack of deep proprioceptive stimulation with continuous body rocking, which is seen as a source of self-comfort. This is often seen in children who are institutionalized and are deprived of mothering and affection.[19]

In young children, social deprivation can lead to developmental failure (psychosocial dwarfism), which is identical to growth hormone deficiency seen in conditions such as pituitary gland damage. When these children are placed in a less hostile and more secure environment, their condition is reversed within a matter of days.[24] In one documented case of maternal deprivation, a 2-year-old child was displaying all the symptoms of severe mental retardation

following a history of lack of care.[19] During the course of her treatment, normal interpersonal stimulation was reintroduced by the therapist. Notably, the early forms of interaction were verbal lulling, tactile stimulation and body rocking. Eventually, with other means of stimulation over a period of a few years, the child was able to overcome her disabilities and develop fully.

In the elderly

A number of studies suggest that there may be a link between lack of physical contact and premature death in the elderly.[8,25,26] One mechanism that has been attributed to the longevity of couples is that social attachment acts as a buffer against stress and anxiety. These findings, coupled with the observation that human contact acts as a regulator of stress, could indicate the importance of physical contact for longevity in adults. However, this statement is highly speculative as it is very difficult to measure lack of physical contact in isolation from social deprivation and detachment. The effects of touch on the elderly are further discussed in the section on the body-self below.

TOUCH AS INTERPERSONAL COMMUNICATION

A handshake, a pat on the shoulder, a gentle stroke and an embrace are all examples of tactile communication, each with its own particular meaning. In some circumstances, touch can be more potent in conveying feelings than can verbal or visual communication.[27] In manual therapy, touch is a potent form of communication that can support the patient's therapeutic process. An example of the use of tactile communication is shown in the treatment of a middle-aged woman who was severely disabled by musculoskeletal injuries. She lost the use of her right arm and was in persistent pain following a complete tear of the rotator cuff muscles during an epileptic seizure. Her condition was further complicated by other painful musculoskeletal conditions that made it difficult for her to walk and sit. At the time I started seeing her, 6 months after her injury, she was severely depressed and expressed a lack of will to live. During her treatment, I extensively used touch to convey messages of support, comfort and reassurance. Her mood change was rapid and dramatic, improving well before her physical symptoms. She seemed to be rarely depressed, was much happier and was often smiling and telling jokes. It is difficult to measure how much the touch element had to do with her psychological improvement. However, I believe that, in this particular case, touch communication was highly significant and was more potent than verbal or visual communication.

TOUCH IN THE DEVELOPMENT OF COMMUNICATION

The root of the potency of touch as a communication modality lies in early childhood. Using tactile and bodily contacts, the baby and mother forge a communication link. The baby evokes a response in the mother, who reciprocates and stimulates the baby in a spiral of communication.[28–31] This spiral may start by a visual or physical cue from the baby, the mother continuing with a tactile response, which the baby answers vocally.[1] This reciprocal communication can be physiological in its nature: the baby's mouth stimulates the mother's nipple, resulting in lactation. This response is, in turn, physically and emotionally comforting to the baby (and the mother). It is believed that these early forms of intimacy and interpersonal communication form templates by which the individual forms subsequent communications and relationships throughout life.[28]

Communication ability matures with the infant's development, and has a sequential progression from a signal type of communication to the more complex development of signs and symbols.[28] Signal communication is received by receptors in the skin conveying immediate sensations such as heat, cold, pain and pleasure.

Although there is a sequential development of communication from tactile signal to abstract sign and symbol, tactile communication is never superseded. The meaning and full significance of many signs and symbols depend on early tactile experiences. To understand the word 'hot' would be virtually impossible without a previous tactile sensation of heat. Frank[28] points out that 'in all symbolic communications such as language, verbal or written, the recipient can decode the message only insofar as his previous experiences provided the necessary meaning and the affective, often sensory, colouring and intensity to give those symbolic messages their content'. Indeed, many words in English (as well as other languages) have a tactile figure of speech to portray emotion, for example 'I am touched', 'I feel', 'I am hurt', which, without previous tactile experiences, would have little meaning.[28]

However, touch remains a primary and potent form of communication throughout life.

Potency of tactile communication

In infants, the potency of tactile communication can be demonstrated when visual communication such as facial expression is compared with tactile stimulation.[32] If, during an interaction between an adult and an infant, the adult keeps a steady, neutral facial expression, the child commonly responds by reducing his or her gaze (at the person), ceasing to smile and possibly even beginning to grimace. However, if in the same expressionless condition, the infant is actively touched by the adult, this response is reduced, even if the touching hand is out of sight.[32]

Tactile communication can be transient, yet its effect on the recipient may reverberate long after the contact has been made. In one study set in a school library, an unsuspecting group of students were touched briefly (for about half a second) while being handed their library card. Once outside the library, this group of students were interviewed and compared with a group of students who were not touched. The 'touch' group reported a positive attitude towards the toucher and the library environment compared with the 'no-touch' group.[33]

TACTILE COMMUNICATION IN THE THERAPEUTIC SETTING

Studies on the effects of touch on the mind and emotions of patients are surprisingly rare in manual therapy, most of the research in this area coming from nursing and psychotherapy. These studies are far from elucidating the nature of touch in a manual therapy setting, but they do provide some insight into the potency of touch as a psychodynamic process.

Therapeutic touch has been shown to be useful during labour, helping to relax women when they did not respond to verbal stimuli.[34] Similarly, touch has been found to be useful in treating individuals suffering from depression and anxiety who did not respond to other forms of communication.[35–37] In counselling, it was found that brief social touch by the therapist facilitated self-exploration by the patient. The touch used in these circumstances was minimal: a handshake, a pat on the shoulder or touching the arm, each lasting only a few seconds.[38] Supportive touch in counselling also promoted a positive evaluation of the counselling by the patient.[39]

Touch is useful in indicating to seriously ill patients that the nurse cares about them. This can be done with a minimum of touch: during one study, the nurse held the patient's wrist while talking. The nurse's touch was perceived by cancer patients to convey confidence, which helped them to cope better with their illness.[41]

The use of touch in a psychiatric ward for selected patients has been shown to increase the patient's verbal interaction, rapport and approach behaviour. In this research, patients who had an aversion to touch were not included in the study. This is a very important point for manual therapists: *some patients may have had negative touch experiences such as sexual or physical abuse and will thus find another person's touch distressing, even in a therapeutic setting.*

INTERPRETATION OF TOUCH

Tactile communication is a complex mixture of the messages being sent and the way in which these messages are understood by the recipient. How touch is interpreted may depend upon the individual's cultural and social background, past experiences, feelings at the time and nature of the patient–therapist relationship (Fig. 15.2).[42] Past touch experiences play an important role in how the patient perceives the manipulation. If the individual has had positive tactile experiences, there are less likely to be complications in deciphering the message's contents. However, negative experiences, such as physical or sexual abuse and touch deprivation, may raise feelings that will negatively influence therapist–patient tactile communication. Body image, areas of taboo and symbolism in the body will also play a part in the interpretation of tactile communication (see below). These different variables will also affect the ability of the giver and recipient to use touch as a form of communication.

Positively, touch can convey messages such as personal acknowledgement, support, intimacy (as in closeness, rather than of a sexual nature)[42–44]

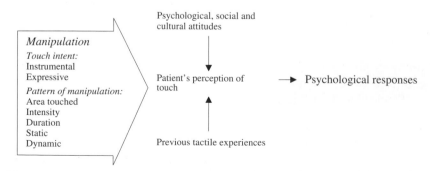

Figure 15.2   Some factors influencing the patient's response to touch.

and reassurance.[32] Touch is experienced as a positive experience when it is perceived as:[43,44]

- appropriate to the situation
- not imposing greater intimacy than the subject desires
- not communicating a negative message.

Negatively, touch may be conveyed or interpreted as aggressive or sexual in nature.[42] This will damage the therapeutic relationship and impede the progression of treatment.

As in other forms of interpersonal communication, there may be misinterpretation of the touch message.[45] Two individuals are involved in the tactile event, each with their own life experiences bearing upon the perception of the tactile messages. For example, misunderstanding could arise from simple differences in the cultural background of patient and therapist.

The relative scarcity of tactile communication in adult life may also be a source for misunderstandings. This 'lack of practice', together with past experiences, can lead to a failure in the ability to use this form of communication, due either to the inability of the giver to send these messages successfully, or to the inability of the recipient to perceive them. For example, some patients will be deeply moved by having supportive touch gently applied to their head (e.g. cranial), whereas, others will be emotionally unmoved by this experience. They will feel the therapist's hand contact with their head, but it has no meaning other than its mechanistic value. Like other forms of communication, the therapist's tactile communication can be developed through awareness and practice.

FEEDBACK AND COMMUNICATION FROM THE PATIENT

So far, tactile communication has been discussed as unidirectional: from therapist to patient. However, during treatment, the patient is continuously responding to the manual event, communicating or 'feeding back' information about the experience of being manipulated (Fig. 15.3).

Spitz observed that communication between mother and child is carried out by means of 'balance, tension (of muscles and other organs), body posture, temperature, vibration, skin and body contact, rhythm, tempo'.[1] Interestingly, this description could have been applied to describe tactile communication during manual treatment. As in the mother–baby communication, patient–therapist cues manifest as changes in muscle tone, facial expression, temperature of the skin, some vocalization and visual contact. These communication cues from the patient are usually very subtle but very important as they help the therapist adjust the technique variables to the patient needs. For example, the amplitude of stretching can be gauged by observing the patient's face and body language. Discomfort or pain caused by treatment will usually be expressed as grimacing, muscle contraction and fine evasive movements. The patients' responses can also indicate how they experience their treatment, for example is their muscle tone reducing, indicating relaxation, or are they still tense, indicating a state of arousal?

TOUCHING THE BODY-SELF IN MANUAL THERAPY

When patients are touched their psyche is also touched; it is virtually impossible to separate the psyche from the body.[46] It is not uncommon to find that a physical treatment may bring about changes in the patient's psychological state, in the form of mood changes, altered perception of body image and behavioural changes. To understand how these changes are brought about, one needs to examine the relationship between the mind and the body, called the *body-self*. The self

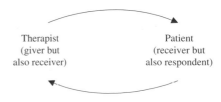

Figure 15.3   Touch and manipulation form bidirectional communication.

is the abstract, the non-physical part of us: mind, emotions, feelings, thoughts, spirituality and the ability to rationalize. The body is the physical part of the self. The body-self has been extensively described in humanistic psychology and philosophy,[47,48] although its definition still remains unresolved. The paradigm chosen here is an adaptation to be used as a working model for manual therapy. In particular, this model will be used to examine the changes in the body-self following physical injury.

The self is dependent on sensory sensations from the body for its nourishment. Marcel[1] writes about this relationship between the self and the body: 'I cannot exactly say that I have a body, but the mysterious link which unites me with my body is the root of my whole potential. The more I am my body, the more of reality is available to me. Things only exist inasmuch as they are in contact with my body and are perceived by it.' Perls, the founder of Gestalt psychotherapy, pointed out that nurturing the body sensation and increasing body awareness can 'feed' the self, promoting integration.[49] Indeed Darbonne,[50] a gestalt therapist and Rolfer, recommends the use of Rolfing to increase body awareness for personal growth. Lowen[51] writes about the feeling of identity that stems from the feeling of contact with the body: 'Without this awareness of bodily feeling and attitudes, a person becomes split into a disembodied spirit and a disenchanted body.' Interestingly, this relationship of the body as nurturing the self can be seen in a pathological condition where the patient is unable to perceive pain. Schilder[52] has observed that such patients are generally insensitive to threatening gestures or dangerous situations, a fundamental behavioural change as a result of altered pain (sensory) perception. A more common situation in which body changes are deeply tied to psychological changes is seen in exercising.[46] Schilder uses dancing as an example of this relationship. He suggests that dancing is one way in which we change the body-self and body image from rigid to loose and flowing: 'the loosening of the body-image will bring with it a particular psychic attitude. Motion thus influences the body-image and leads from a change in the body-image to a change in psychic attitude.'[52]

Jung[50] also sees spirituality as stemming from body processes: 'If we reconcile ourselves with the mysterious truth that spirit is the living body seen from within and the body is the outer manifestation of the living spirit, the two being really one, then we can understand why it is that the attempt to transcend the present level of consciousness must give its due to the body. We shall also see that belief in the spirit cannot tolerate an outlook that denies the body.'

BODY IMAGE AND SYMBOLISM IN THE BODY

Body image is how a person sees their physical self in their mind's eye.[53] Body image consists of the external envelope of the body and the body's internal volume or space (Fig. 15.4).[54] This physical extent of the body is called the *body boundaries*. The relationship of an individual to

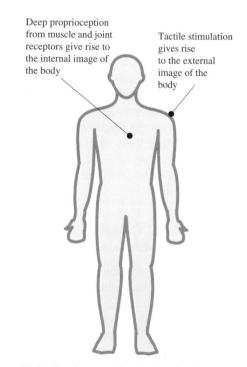

Deep proprioception from muscle and joint receptors give rise to the internal image of the body

Tactile stimulation gives rise to the external image of the body

Figure 15.4 The image of the body-self arises from sensory feedback.

others and objects around the body is called the *body space*.[54]

The perception of the envelope of the body arises from the skin combined with visual information.Vision tends to dominate proprioception, especially with respect to the external appearance of the body. Deeper or volume body image arises from the deep proprioceptors of the body (receptors in the muscles and joints). These also provide a sense of the physical extent of movement, for example how far one can bend or lift. Motion and physical activities are therefore important ingredients in the formation and maintenance of the body image. These sensory experiences are heavily modulated by the mind and psychological processes. They form a body image that is somewhat different from physical reality.[55] Both body image and its symbolisms are dynamic rather than static perceptions, changing with movement, posture, different emotional states, our relationship to others and objects (such as clothing) and also in time, with ageing and different life experiences.[47,52,54–56] Because these perceptions are dynamic, manual therapy can also be a catalyst for a change in the way the patient perceives his or her body.

Box 15.1 gives some examples of exercises in body image, particularly images arising from proprioception.

Touching the symbolic body

Within the complex of body image, the individual will also symbolically label different parts of the body to give them internal, personal meanings. For example, the back may be related to being able to carry 'life's burdens'. It is the part that holds us physically and emotionally upright, and when we feel the need for support, we search for a 'back-up'. Indeed when someone becomes a burden, you tell them to 'get off my back'. Alternatively, you may refer to them as being 'a pain in the neck'. This process can be used to

---

Box 15.1   Introspection exercise for body image

Perception of the outer surface of the body
Closing the eyes and without movement, the contact of the skin is very vague. The skin is not perceived as a smooth continuous sheath but rather a blurred surface which is merging with the outside world (Schilder 1964.[51]). However, when the eyes are open the outline of the hand is very sharp and clearly differentiated from the space around the body. When we touch an object with our eyes shut, we first feel the object and only with further introspection can we feel our skin. If you look at your hand and then close your eyes the sensation from the skin or the envelope of the body seems to be deeper than what you see.

Distinct sensations of the skin are felt when the skin is in direct contact with external objects. If you introspect feeling the forearm there will be a very blurred, a discontinued image of the skin. If you now touch your forearm with your other hand or an object the skin will take a distinct shape. If you now rub the hand or the object across the forearm the shape of the forearm becomes even more acute. If you compare both forearms in your mind's eye, you will be more aware of the touched forearm, it will feel more continuous and distinct. This imprint may last for quite some time.

Perception of the internal space/volume of the body
If you contract the muscles of your whole arm and compare it with the relaxed arm, the tense arm will feel heavier and its volume more clear.

With your eyes shut, slowly open and close the fist of one hand, and compare it with the relaxed non-moving hand. The non-moving hand will feel blurred and indistinct. The moving hand will feel voluminous, distinct and clearly delineated from the surrounding space. The stronger the force of contraction the clearer and more defined the internal volume and the outline of the hand.

Perception of the centre mass of the body
As you hold this book it will feel as if the lower part of the book which is closer to your hand is heavier than the top of the book, as if all its weight has accumulated at the bottom leaving the top empty. Similarly we conceive our centre of gravity: when we stand the feet feel heaviest and diminishing upward. When lying down or sitting the part in contact with the supporting surface feels heavier and the parts further away lighter and more empty. Interestingly when lifting an arm or a leg the perceived centre of mass is somewhere in the centre of the limb very close to the true physical centre of mass; when we move our limb we do not think of the different limb segments of joints or muscles. This could be important in rehabilitating the motor system: to rehabilitate the whole limb rather then individual segments.

look at virtually every anatomical structure in the body, including internal organs, for example to love with the heart or to fear with the gut. Even muscles can have symbolic meanings. Nathan[57] perceptively writes about the functions and symbolism of the biceps muscles: 'flex the elbow joint, supinate the elbow joint, help stabilise the shoulder joint, raise a stiff sash window, lift my glass of beer every evening, use a tenon saw every day, shake my fist – express an emotion, attract (some) women, win weight lifting competitions frequently'.

In injury and illness, the symbolic part of the body may change. This may lead to negative changes in perception, symbolism and the feelings of the individual towards the damaged area of the body. For example, if the back symbolizes the ability to carry life's burdens, spinal injury may shatter this image, leading to anxiety and fear. The effect of treatment in this situation is not limited to mechanically fixing the spine but also encompasses reinstating its psychological symbolism.

DEVELOPMENT OF THE BODY-SELF AND BODY IMAGE

Body image seems to develop in parallel with sensory and motor development.[52] Early tactile and proprioceptive stimulation in the womb, infancy and childhood provide the stimulation and basis for the development of the body-self.[58] The maturation of proprioception is completed before that of other sensory faculties. This gives the developing fetus and young infant its first 'taste' of the body-self compared with the non-self (the world around us).[59,60] Schilder[52] writes about early tactile influences: 'The touches of others, the interest others take in the different parts of our body, will be of enormous importance in the development of the postural model of the body.' Kulka[29] suggests that movement helps the infant to develop a deep internal sense of the self, a body image which goes beyond the skin. Freud[51] writes about the importance of tactile stimulation for the development of the ego (the self): 'The ego is ultimately derived from bodily sensations, chiefly from those springing from the surface of the body. It may thus be regarded as a mental projection of the surface of the body'.

This process has a parallel in embryonic development. The nervous system and skin arise from the same embryonic tissue – the ectoderm – which forms the covering of the embryo. During development, a part of the ectoderm turns in on itself to differentiate into the nervous system.[61] What remains on the outside becomes the sense organs: skin (tactile), vision, hearing, taste and smell. Montagu sees the nervous system as being a buried part of the skin, or alternatively the skin being an exposed portion of the nervous system: 'the external nervous system'.[61] Following birth, with the development of sight, vision together with other sensory modalities will play an important role in forming the body image, in particular the external appearance of the body. However, proprioception remains an important source of body image, throughout the life of the individual.

If proprioceptive stimulation is not available in early life, it may lead to a basic distortion and lack of perception in the formation of the body-self.[62] For example, such deprivation is believed to occur in child autism. Positively, touch can be nurturing to the well-being of the body-self image; however, abusive touch can lead to a pathological perception of the body-self.

THE BODY-SELF AND BODY IMAGE: DISUNITY, FRAGMENTATION AND DISTORTION

In the ideal situation, the body and self are one: the body-self. If you are engrossed in reading this book, you might be oblivious to the existence of, say, your arm or even the rest of your body. You can be said to have unity between the body and the self. If you now concentrate on your arm, a paradox arises: you have a self-body disunity. Your self is now in the position of looking down at your body. This disunity is normal and transient; by the next paragraph you will probably have again become unaware of your arm. If, however, while reading, your back begins to hurt or your arms are getting tired holding the book, you will become progressively aware of the pain. The disunity is now constant and has a biologically protective function: to warn that you are stressing your body, signalling the need for a change of position. The self is being called upon to observe the distressed body. If, for some reason, your pain is chronic, the disunity will also become continuous. A protective function is now becoming a fragmenting experience.

Health and well-being are often associated with a physical sensation of the body as a whole. When all is working well, the body and the self are a unified whole (Fig. 15.5). In physical or psychological ill-health, this unity is fragmented: from unity of the body-self to a state of disunity, in which the injured part becomes segregated from the rest of the body. The simplest example is when the external envelope, the skin, is cut, resulting in discontinuation of the body image. This fragmentation of body image can go beyond

the skin and occur in 'deeper' structures. For example, a chronically painful knee can be psychologically 'encapsulated in attention', with a loss of sense of continuity in the limb. A simple exercise is to compare a painful with a non-painful side of your body (for example, the painful side of your neck with the other). If you scan with your mind's eye the non-painful side of the body from head to foot, the scanning process will be continuous and uninterrupted. However, if you scan your painful side, you will notice that this process tends to get stuck or interrupted at the site of pain, so the sense of continuity is lost.

Pain can have a profound effect on body-self and body image. It brings into focus an area which before injury was a part of the whole. In these circumstances, the patient's response is to segregate the injured part from the rest of the body. Indeed, the patient who has neck tension will often describe the symptom as 'the neck is painful', indicating a disassociation of the neck with 'its' pain from the self. He may be unaware that the tension in his shoulder is something he does to himself in response to a stressful experience.[17] Segregation has different perceptual forms: it is an imaging process in which the damaged area is either being focused on and enlarged, diminished or totally excluded from the body image (Fig. 15.6). Patients whose damaged part is perceived to be out of proportion are dominated by their pain. Their condition permeates every facet of their life, affecting their physical activities and psychological well-being. This abnormal relationship may not be proportional to the extent of injury or the level of pain the patient is feeling. Other patients deal with pain by a process of diminution: their body schema of the damaged part becomes smaller or even distant. They will often say, for example, 'I have a high threshold of pain', and may even go to the extent of abolishing that part of the body from their mind's eye.

Some patients will project their own fragmentation process to the therapist, who is encouraged to perceive them as a disunited entity. They often expect the damaged part to be treated in isolation from the rest of the body and their life processes. Nathan[57] suggests that, if it were

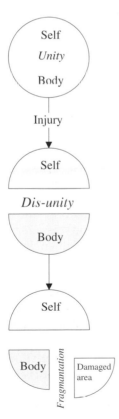

Figure 15.5 Unity, disunity and fragmentation in the body-self.

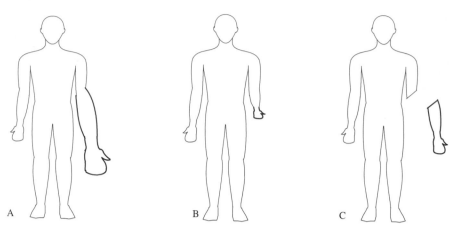

Figure 15.6   Following injury or illness, the patient's body-self image may be distorted in several ways. (A) The perception of the damaged area may increase and dominate the patient's body-self and life. (B) The damaged area may be diminished in the body-self image, the patient choosing to be unaware of it. (C) The patient may totally segregate the damaged area from the rest of the healthy body.

possible, the patient would leave the body with the therapist, to be collected at the end of treatment. The patient's notions can also affect the actual physical elements of manipulation. The patient may urge the therapist to take away the discomfort and pain by demanding a harder and deeper manipulation. This body-self disunity by the patient is well symbolized by Wilber,[63] who sees the disunity in ourselves as a horseman (the self) riding on a horse (the body): 'I beat it or praise it, I feed and clean and nurse it when necessary. I urge it on without consulting it and I hold it back against its will. When my body-horse is well-behaved I generally ignore it, but when it gets unruly – which is all too often – I pull out the whip to beat it back into reasonable submission.' This analogy well portrays the clinical situation in which the patient perceives the therapist as a 'therapeutic whip' that will beat the disobedient part of the body back into health and unity.

Abnormal relationships between the self and the body may take place in mental illness or psychological conditions. Lowen[50] points out that abnormal body perception can be observed in schizophrenic patients who have a 'loss of touch' with their body and therefore with reality. In anorexia-bulimia and depression the patient may have a disassociation with the body.[56] In patients suffering from depression, this may result in the infliction of self-pain to increase body awareness or a sense of reality.

NURTURING AND REINTEGRATION OF THE BODY-SELF BY MANUAL THERAPY

Manual therapy can potentially be a catalyst for processes such as increasing body awareness, highlighting body boundaries and body space, and integrating the body-self. The physical interactions of early life form the foundations of the body-self and body image. The potency of manual therapy in influencing body-self processes in adult life is partly derived from these early life experiences. Manipulation is also a rich source of sensory stimulation that can be available for the therapeutic nourishment of the body-self. Examples of the integrative potency of touch/manipulation are shown in Figure 15.7.

Various forms of manipulation will influence the body-self processes in different ways. Techniques that stimulate skin receptors, such as massage, can be used to reinforce the sense of the body's envelope. Passive technique can provide awareness of the internal space of the

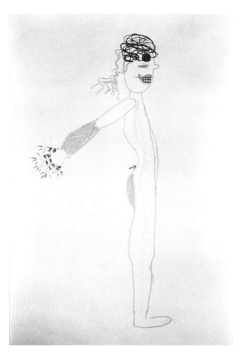

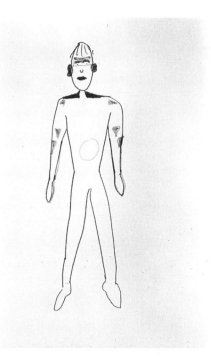

A *Subject 1* Before a manual experience. An example of how pain and discomfort may dominate the body-image. The main focus was the forearm and hands which were aching before treatment.

B *Subject 1* After a manual experience. The subject had less tension and discomfort in the arms, which had a more balanced representation in the body image.

Figure 15.7   The integrative potential of touch. During a workshop in therapeutic touch, participants were asked to draw their body-image before and after a touch/manipulation experience. The treatment given was according to the drawings and feedback from the subject. After the treatment the subjects were asked to draw their body again. The drawing served to highlight the changes in the subject's body experience and body-image after a touch/manual event. (Photographs courtesy of The Centre for Professional Development in Osteopathy and Manual Therapy, London.)

limb and the quality and extent of movement, as well as of the connectedness and relationship of different body parts to each other.[55] Active techniques, in which the patient is voluntarily contracting or moving against resistance, can give a sense of the inside space of the body or a sense of strength, or highlight areas of weakness. In areas of the body where the patient may feel weak, active techniques can be used to give a feeling of internal support, strength and continuity.[55] The physical interaction of the therapist with the patient during active techniques has a strong psychological effect, one which is unlikely to occur during physical activity performed with objects such as weights.

An example of when I have used passive techniques is in a case of a patient who was suffering from severe repetitive strain injury. This condition made him disproportionately aware of the palms of his hand in relation to other parts of his body, his palms totally dominating his body image and daily activities. Part of the treatment was to 'resize' the palms to their preinjury proportions in the body schema, and to give a sense of continuity to the whole upper part of his body and arms. To integrate the envelope of the body schema I used massage and stroking techniques over the whole upper limbs and torso, with only minor attention to the palms. Deeper integration of the internal volume and extent of movement was achieved by passive whole-limb movement and active techniques. During the active techniques, the whole arm and torso were used, the hand taking only a

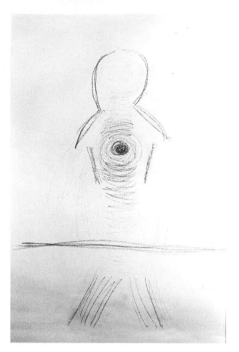

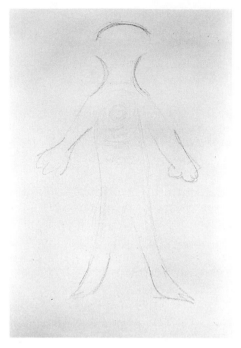

C *Subject 2* Before a manual experience. There is a split between the upper and lower body, and the arms, hands and feet are not represented in the body image.

D *Subject 2* After a manual experience. There is more integration in the body; the upper-lower body split has disappeared, and the arms, hands and feet are now represented in the body image.

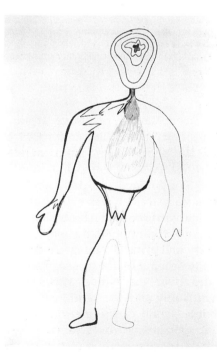

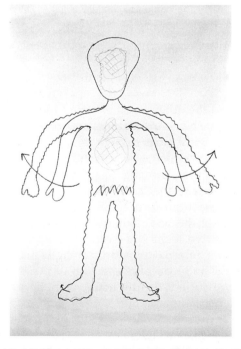

E *Subject 3* Before a manual experience. Notice the head to body relationship. The subject described the head as being enclosed in a walnut. There is left–right and upper–lower body imbalance.

F *Subject 3* After a manual experience. There is a better balance and integration of the head and body, and between the left and right sides of the body. The arrows on the drawing depict a sensation of fine involuntary movement within the body.

proportional role in the movement, i.e. being integrated into the total movement pattern. Usually, following treatment, the patient would remark that he was now more aware of the whole upper part of his body and less focused on his hands.

A situation in which I have used an active technique was in a case of a patient who reported that his arms felt 'disconnected' from the rest of his body. Following the use of active techniques for the upper limbs and chest area, the patient reported that this type of manipulation helped him to feel the arms as being a part of his body. In another case, a patient came for postural advice. He was holding his head with his chin protruding forward, causing increased lordosis of the cervical spine. This posture was apparently related to his adolescence when he was ashamed of the size of his chest, so compensated for it posturally. He had little awareness of how to bring his head to the correct position and there was a sense that he had little control of his posterior neck muscles. I used active techniques such as dynamic neck extensions to make him aware of these muscles. With these techniques, the patient was able to move with more ease into the correct position. This postural awareness was not present during guidance techniques. This case is, of course, multivariate as there were many layers to the patient's posture and his body-self image. It is used to highlight only one facet of the treatment relating to deep proprioception, which is highly facilitated during active–dynamic techniques (see Section 2). With this patient, active techniques were also being used psychologically to empower an area that the patient felt was weak.

In mental illness and psychological conditions in which disassociation with the body is present, touch has been used to promote a sense of self and identity in relation to the patient's current situation and space. The influence of touch on the individual's sense of self has also been called 'reality orientating'.[64] For example, in Scandinavia, Body Awareness Therapy is practised by physiotherapists in the treatment of psychotic conditions such as schizophrenia.[65] One of the stated aims is to help these patients to reintegrate by the use of body awareness exercise as well as massage.

Although body awareness seems to be necessary for the positive change towards body-self integration, there exists a paradox in this approach. Initially, self-awareness may increase the disunity in the body-self as the self 'decides' to observe (introspect) the body with heightened concentration. In some individuals, heightened awareness may be a negative process that amplifies disunity rather than promoting unity. Obsession with body awareness is often seen in neurosis and hypochrondriasis, in which individuals are totally absorbed by the activities of their body.[47,66]

Self-image in the elderly

In the elderly, the body-self image is changing in a negative direction as many structures and functions of the body are diminishing or beginning to fail. The deterioration in body image can be further exacerbated by lack of social and physical contact.[67] Isolation may be exacerbated by the failure of other sensory modalities such as hearing or sight.

Touch is very important for the elderly as it breaks through the isolation, providing human contact with all its psychological implications: support, comfort, compassion and a positive stimulus for the self-image.[67]

PLEASURE AND PAIN IN MANUAL THERAPY

Pleasure is a very important therapeutic tool for personal integration and healing. Lowen[67] writes about pleasure and its integrative qualities: 'Since the primary needs of an organism have to do with the maintenance of its integrity, pleasure is associated with the sense of well-being that arises when this integrity is assured. In its simplest form pleasure reflects the healthy operation of the vital processes of the body.' Lowen sees pleasure and pain as opposites on a spectrum (Fig. 15.8). Pain gives rise to muscular contraction, withdrawal and fragmentation of

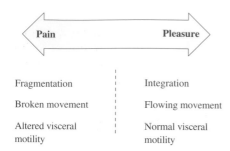

Figure 15.8 The pain–pleasure spectrum in relation to the body-self.

the body-self. It makes movements abrupt and jerky and may alter autonomic motility of vital organs,[65] like breath-holding, increased heart rate or the nauseous feelings associated with pain. Pleasure can be seen as the opposite, promoting expansion and integration.[69] It encourages normal flow in movement and autonomic motility, both of which are important for normal healing and well-being.

MANIPULATION AS A SOURCE OF PLEASURE

One common 'side-effect' of manual therapy is physical pleasure, a positive element of treatment that encourages expansion, integration and a sense of well-being. It should be promoted rather then actively suppressed during treatment. There are two forms of pleasure that can be derived from manipulation:

1. Manual treatment can be in itself a source of tactile pleasure.
2. The return to health, well-being and normal functioning of a part or all of the body is pleasurable, as seen for example, when a muscle returns to normal function following an injury or when health returns after an illness.

Stimulation of deep proprioceptors provides internal pleasure: the pleasure of muscle effort in active techniques; the sensation of full joint movement in passive techniques; the pleasure of muscles and joints being stretched. This is very similar to the pleasure experienced during physical activities, for example that of muscles being

stretched in yoga, the inner body space in Tai-Chi, the exhilarating sense of muscle effort in running and the joy of dancing.[45]

The pleasure of movement can be traced to early childhood. Movement such as crawling, rolling, sitting and handling objects, is usually executed with obvious pleasure.[29,52] Kulka[29] hypothesized that the infant's active movement is a means of expression and a release of tension. Motor urges, are described as having the same cyclical quality as other bodily urges, such as oral, excretory and genital.[46] Pleasure and satisfaction are achieved when the individual follows this urgency by movement and completes the tension–release cycle. Later, as the child matures, the movement urges become highly organized into such physical activities as sports and play.[29]

PAIN, PLEASURE AND PLEASURABLE OR THERAPEUTIC PAIN

Patients very often ask to be manipulated very forcefully, deeply and painfully, yet derive pleasure from being physically hurt. This phenomenon is termed 'pleasurable pain' or 'therapeutic pain'. There may be several reasons for the need to be physically hurt during treatment. One may be related to the close anatomical organization of the punishment and pleasure centres in the brain. Activity in one area may spread to the adjacent areas, resulting in blurring of boundaries, pain being experienced as pleasurable. This can be experienced by pressing with one hand on the other forearm, slowly building the pressure. There is initially a pleasant pressure sensation, which will gradually turn into pain as the pressure increases. However, the pleasure of pressure may still be there, mixed with the sensation of pain.

There may be also psychological and social origins of the need for painful treatment. A common and normal pattern of human behaviour is to make sacrifices to an ultimate goal. An individual will often endure pain because at the end there is a promise of pleasure and well-being. For example, when one gets a muscle cramp or stiffness, the natural inclination is to stretch the painful muscle, a process which is in itself painful but promises the termination of pain and the pleasure of the muscle returning to normal function. In such circumstances, it is not pain one is seeking but rather the end result, which is pleasure.[68] A variation on pain-seeking patterns is seen in patients who view pain as a price for healing – the 'no pain, no gain' belief. Some patients believe that pain holds redemption. For the treatment to be effective, it must also be painful: 'I have damaged myself, it is due to life's excesses and I will redeem myself through pain' (as in religious redemption for the fakir). These patients seek a painful treatment and may be more tolerant of pain.

Pain during treatment may also serve the patient's physical and psychological needs to be met. This type of contact may be seen in patients who are remote from physical, bodily sensations. In some, this need can be only satisfied at the point near structural rupture. Some patients may feel that, by working deeply and directly at the source of damage, the therapist has found the 'source of all evils' and is about to expel it from the body. In such circumstances, a gentle treatment may be perceived as the inability of the therapist to find the source of pain or cure it.

At the extreme end of pain-seeking lie those with masochistic tendencies, which may be associated with the early tactile relationship of the parent with child.[37] In these individuals, states of neither pleasure nor pain can be sustained or satisfied: they are permanently seeking the other extreme. The patient's masochistic tendencies must not be fed in treatment as they may develop into abuse and will not serve as a reparative, healing process for the individual.

Pleasurable pain, such as during stretching, deep pressure or massage, can be used with those patients who 'demand' a strong treatment but not with those who reject such treatment or have injuries for which a forceful treatment is contraindicated. Even if a forceful treatment is used, pain should be on the pleasurable rather than the severely painful side. *Pain for the purpose of pain is non-therapeutic*, but treatment that involves some pain may sometimes be inevitable. 'Negative' pain, which is sharp, bruising, hot or tearing in nature, should be avoided. These types of pain are probably non-therapeutic and are indicators that the manipulation is excessive and is causing further damage.

MANIPULATION, PAIN, PLEASURE AND REINTEGRATION

Evoking a sense of pleasure from the damaged area is also important for the integration process. A pleasurable treatment can promote 'opening-up', a positive sense of the body and reintegration. The pattern and extent of touch are very important for reinstating continuity in the body. Working on a wider area than the injury and introducing pleasure may help the patient to reintegrate the injured area with the surrounding healthy tissues. This pattern of touching can be often seen when someone is hurt: he or she will tend to rub the painful and the surrounding tissue vigorously as if to re-blend the damaged with the healthy tissues (vibration of the skin may also gate the pain signals). Treatment that causes pain should end with a diffuse and pleasant pattern, as manipulation that is localized and painful will increase the focus on the damaged area, promoting further segregation, rejection and contraction of the painful ('ill') area.

Pleasure can be seen as a positive feedback for the patient from an area that has been a source of negative sensations. When any part of the body is in pain, there may be a need to disown the area or reject it from the body. A treatment that evokes sensations of pleasure from an injured and painful part may help the patient to feel like reowning that part of the body. I often see this in my practice. For example, a patient complained of 20 years of neck and shoulder pain, her attitude toward her neck and shoulder being negative and rejectionist. The first treatment incorporated gentle, broad soft-tissue massage and stretching, with an emphasis on creating a sense of pleasure from an area that had always been a source of pain. At the end of treatment, the patient's attitude was dramatically changed. She was now positive about that part of her body, gently stroking it rather than poking it deeply as she had done prior to treatment. She was now talking about the pleasant tingling sensation in her neck and shoulder. This I see as the first step towards the process of integration and healing.

TACTILE CONTACT: EROTIC OR THERAPEUTIC?

In classical psychology (e.g. Freud),[52] tactile pleasure (or any other pleasure) is associated with eroticism. This view has been challenged by such people as Boyesen,[70] who put forward the concept of non-sexual sensory pleasure. Indeed, it is very difficult to imagine that all touch is erotic in nature. Non-erotic pleasure can be seen in all our other senses:[71] The visual pleasure of seeing something aesthetically pleasing; the pleasure of hearing music; the pleasure of smelling a flower or tasting Belgian chocolates; and, along these lines, the pleasure of being touched.

However, there are problems with tactile pleasure. Generally, the most pleasurable of tactile experiences is another person's touch. Furthermore, in adulthood, there may be a strong association between touch and erotic pleasure. This association may spill into treatment, with both the giver and the receiver misinterpreting touch as being sexual. This may be further complicated by taboo areas in the body that have greater sexual symbolism and are prohibited for touch outside intimate contact (see below). Treatment of these areas may be perceived to be erotic. For example, the sensuality associated with the pelvis being touched will be different from that of touching the patient's elbow. To overcome this problem, the therapist–patient contract must be very clear in stating the treatment boundaries. It must state where touch will be applied and its therapeutic purpose. The intention of the therapist must be also clear: pleasure is to be used solely for therapeutic purposes and does not contain sexual messages. This principle of intent is discussed below.

Some patients may use manual therapy to fulfil their needs for tactile pleasure and physical/social contact. This does not necessarily arise from erotic needs but has been previously described as an instinctive and psychological need for well-being. Morris[2] points out that, in some circumstances, the manual therapist's role in society is to provide a substitute for lack of touch in relationships. An individual may seek to fill this void by seeking a substitute physical contact.[72,73] In this case, 'professional touchers' such as manual therapists fulfil the needs of the seeker for body contact. This is carried out in an environment in which the patient feels safe from the erotic connotations of tactile pleasure.

Aversion to pleasure

Although it has been advocated that pleasure should be seen as a positive element in treatment, some individuals may have an aversion to pleasure and may find pleasurable touch unbearable. This may result from an association of tactile pleasure with eroticism, which they are trying to suppress.[54] In this group of patients, pleasure elicited during treatment may provoke a state of anxiety and fear.

TABOO AREAS OF THE BODY

Not all areas of the body have the same emotional 'weight,' and the patient's response may therefore differ according to the area manipulated. There seems to be an agreement in human studies about which areas of the body are more emotionally 'charged' (Fig. 15.9). The more 'charged' an area is, the more the patient may feel insecure, anxious, threatened and aroused when the area is touched.

In general, extensor surfaces are less emotive or intimate than flexor areas of the body. Indeed, the least emotive or taboo areas are the back of the forearms and the shoulders.[74] 'Ventral taboo' is commonly observed in manual therapy, treatment often being confined to dorsal surfaces such as the back (spine) or extensor surfaces of the limbs. Ventral surfaces of the body are manipulated less often.

Orifices have the highest taboo value in society.[2,37,75] These areas include the genitals, breasts, mouth, ears, eyes and nostrils. This taboo extends well into manual therapy. Even if it is

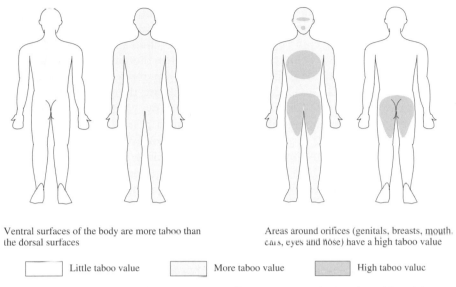

Ventral surfaces of the body are more taboo than
the dorsal surfaces

Areas around orifices (genitals, breasts, mouth,
ears, eyes and nose) have a high taboo value

☐ Little taboo value   ☐ More taboo value   ▨ High taboo value

Figure 15.9   Taboo areas of the human body (figures represent both male and female).

clear, for example, that the pelvic floor needs direct manual work, it is often recommended that such manipulation should be performed in the presence of a third party in the room (to reduce intimacy and for medicolegal reasons).

There may be also some difference between the limbs and the trunk in the level of unease on part of the patient. The trunk seems to represent the individual's core, where the primary identity of the self is concentrated.[76] Touching the trunk may therefore elicit more anxiety than touching the limbs. However, one of the least intrusive forms of touch is to pat someone's back.[74] Another area of taboo is the head. In adult life, the head is rarely touched. In contrast, young children often have their heads touched or ruffled by adults. This could be important to therapists who use cranial techniques: touching the patient's head may initiate an emotional release. Indeed, it is not unusual to evoke strong emotions when the head is handled.

In manual therapy, the contract between the patient and the practitioner should clearly define the use of touch, and that touch may extend to taboo areas of the body. To avoid misinterpretation, as part of the introduction of my work to the patient I make it very clear that I will be using my hands for the treatment (as a

surprising number of patients may be unaware that touch will be used during their osteopathic session). Furthermore, whenever I need to work on a taboo area of the body, such as the anterior ribs in female patients, I will always inform them of what I am about to do, state its purpose and ask permission to apply my hands to that area of their body.

THERAPEUTIC MANIPULATION

The human touch has a therapeutic quality, with the capacity to influence whole-person processes. However, not all touch or manipulation events contain a therapeutic quality. This chapter examines what makes touch therapeutic and, in particular, how therapists can develop the therapeutic qualities of their touch.

ORIGINS OF TOUCH-HEALING

The biological and psychological mechanisms that 'tie' touch in with therapeutic processes have two origins. One is the individual's feelings and the association made between manipulation and healing in relation to earlier life experiences. The other is that touch has an instinctive healing capacity not directly related to the individual's previous experiences. The quality and meaning of touch, as well as the need to give and receive touch, changes with different developmental stages.[77] Comforting touch given to a child is different from therapeutic touch given to an adult, there being, for example, a marked difference between a parent comforting a child after a fall and a nurse's comforting touch of an adult patient. However, there may be some similarities (see below).

Association between touch and healing can be traced back to the early attachment behaviour of the infant to the mother, in which touch and tactile stimulation play an important part in bonding. This relationship begins in the womb in a primitive form, becoming a more complex attachment behaviour from the moment of birth and over the first few years of life. In the womb, kinesthetic and tactile stimulation provides early sensations that are associated with security and support.[29] Following birth, when the baby is placed on its mother's body and suckling is initiated, the comfort and security of intrauterine life is extended into the outside world. During the first year of life the baby is totally reliant on the mother for all its needs.[20] When the baby is in distress, be it emotional or physical, the mother will soothe it by holding, gentle stroking or massage. This physical comforting behaviour is continued throughout childhood. When the child falls or is physically hurt, the parent will stroke the skin over the injured area, kiss it better or hold the child.[78] Most parents discover that, when their child is hurt, no measure of verbal comfort will stop the child crying, unless physical contact is made and the child is hugged or kissed. It has been shown that verbal comfort is not sufficient to calm distressed hospitalized children, but when tactile comfort is added, it has a more potent calming effect.[78] The comforting touch and the encouragement help the child to achieve not just emotional well-being, but also a more effective physiological balance. Reite,[8] who studied the effects of touch, attachment and health in primates, proposes that 'touch can be viewed as a signal stimulus capable of evoking or reactivating a more complex organismic reaction, one component of which is improved physiological functioning.'

As the child grows older (from about 11 to 13 years old), there is generally less physical contact with the parents.[6,37,77] This decrease in contact is also seen in 'therapeutic' touch. There are obviously many variations in the amount of touch that takes place during these years, depending on, for example, culture, education and social status. During these years, there is generally little comforting touch, and the little there is comes largely from individuals outside the close family circle. The quality of touch during this period also changes and does not resemble the comforting touch of early childhood. Probably the only touch that has a therapeutic quality is that provided by health professionals such as doctors, nurses or manual therapists. This skilled therapeutic touch has a precise, limited purpose and only occurs for specific needs. It does not replace or imitate the parental comforting touch.

Comforting touch in adult life is mostly given by the individual's partner or friends. The need for skilled therapeutic touch is met by various health practitioners and, increasingly, by a vast range of manual therapists (in massage, osteopathy, physiotherapy, aromatherapy, chiropractic, shiatsu, etc.). Although the need for comforting contact tends to reduce in adulthood, there may be a reversion to the tactile needs of early life in situations of danger, incapacity, anxiety, bereavement and illness.[37,79] Perhaps, in the same way as the parent's touch can soothe the helplessness of the child, therapeutic touch in adult life can support healing and well-being.[37] Reite[8] states, 'The strong belief that touch has healing powers may be related to the fact that, having once been a major component in the development of attachment bonds, it retains the ability to act as a releaser of certain physiological accompaniments of attachment – specifically, those associated with good feelings states and good health.'

Although the relationship between touch and healing may be a learning experience, as the association may imply, the attachment behaviour between the mother and her child and their physical contact patterns are partly genetic/instinctive in origin,[6] and partly learned from previous experiences such as those of the mother as an infant herself.[23] These patterns stem from the same instinctive behaviour seen in parenting (sometimes called care-taking behaviour).[6] This implies that the need for receiving (therapeutic) touch may be at some level an instinctive pattern of behaviour during physical and emotional distress (similar behaviour being seen in other primates). Indeed, Bowlby[6] points out that this behaviour in adults is not regressive: 'in sickness and calamity, adults often become demanding of others; in conditions of sudden danger or disaster a person will almost certainly seek proximity to another known and trusted person. In such circumstances an increase in attachment behavior is recognised by all as natural. It is therefore extremely misleading for the epithet "regressive" to be applied to every manifestation of attachment behavior in adult life.' He further adds, 'to dub attachment behavior in adult life regressive is indeed to overlook the vital role that it plays in the life of man from cradle to the grave.'

THERAPEUTIC INTENT

Different conditions require different therapeutic intents, and matching the therapeutic intent with the patient's condition is essential for a successful treatment outcome. Intent has physical manifestations that will affect the way in which the therapist touches the patient. One case that can help to demonstrate the importance of this matching is the case of a young woman who complained of severe and diffuse back pain. Her symptoms had started a few months before, and I initially related the injury to her work, in which she occasionally had to lift boxes. On examination of her back, there was severe and diffuse muscle tenderness spanning the lumbar to cervical spine. No other pathological changes were found. Interestingly, the patient was chaperoned by a member of her family, who used to sit in the room throughout the course of treatment. During the first four treatments, the patient received a mechanistic massage and articulatory techniques for her back and neck (as

described in Section 1). However, she was only receiving transient relief from her pain. On the fifth treatment date, she came alone for treatment. I used that occasion to enquire whether there were currently any events in her life that could be a source of stress. She responded by breaking down, crying and becoming highly distressed. It emerged that her parents had arranged for her to be married to a complete stranger, which had placed her under severe emotional stress. From then on, the course, aims and choice of technique changed dramatically. She was immediately referred for counselling, and at the same time the treatment changed from a mechanical 'fix it' treatment to supportive and relaxing treatment. The change in her symptoms was dramatic thereafter, most of her back and neck pain disappearing by the second treatment. What started as a direct, curative treatment aimed at spinal muscles and joints was transformed into a therapeutic whole-person healing process. In this case, failure to match intent with the patient's condition resulted in ineffective treatment. Only when the right intent was introduced did a positive change in the patient's health take place. The differences between the two therapeutic events can be analysed by grouping manipulation and touch into two forms of intent:[74]

1. *Instrumental manipulation*: which aims mechanically to cure or prevent the progression of the patient's condition.
2. *Expressive manipulation*: accepting the patient as a whole – body and mind – with the aim of curing or preventing the progression of the patient's condition as a whole-person process.

INSTRUMENTAL AND EXPRESSIVE MANIPULATION

The aim of instrumental touch is to, *mechanically* and by direct contact with the damaged tissues, cure, repair or prevent progression of the condition.[76] The hands of the therapist are the therapeutic tools, just as a scalpel is for a surgeon. By the mechanistic use of these tools, the therapist is attempting to 'correct' a 'mechanical failure' in the patient's structure or affect local tissue physiology. To stretch a shortened tissue mechanically or to increase blood flow through an ischaemic muscle can be considered to be a mechanistic approach. Instrumental manipulation is also used in carrying out diagnostic procedures such as examining the range of movement of a joint. It can generally be said that instrumental manipulation is biomechanical in its intent. The use of instrumental techniques is often associated with the view of the body as a mechanical entity separated from the self.[57]

The aim of expressive manipulation is to support total body healing and self-regulation processes. Expressive touch acknowledges the person as a whole: a body-self entity. Expressive manipulation involves awareness and empathy with the feelings and emotional state of the patient.[80] One of the most important principles in expressive manipulation is that *the contents of the manual messages are formed mainly by the therapist's intentions and only to lesser extent by the physical elements of the technique*. In expressive manipulation the technique becomes the vehicle for the therapist's intention. Differences between instrumental and expressive manipulation can be illustrated by looking at two common clinical conditions: a patient suffering from a painful neck due to emotional stress and a patient suffering from a musculoskeletal injury such as an ankle sprain. Treatment of an ankle sprain will be largely instrumental, biomechnical in character, with the involvement of only a hint of expressive touch. In this case, instrumental manipulation may consist of joint articulation to facilitate local repair of periarticular structures. In contrast, the patient who is suffering from neck pain will require an expressive form of treatment, low on mechanical or instrumental elements. In this condition, a supportive and relaxing form of manipulation is more appropriate. In a psychosomatic condition such as this, using an instrumental intent may fail to meet the patient's emotional needs. Equally, treating a musculoskeletal injury solely using expressive manipulation will fail to stimulate local tissue repair mechanisms. The differences between expressive and instrumental manipulation are further summarized in Figure 15.10.

It is advocated that a pragmatic approach should be used when correlating therapeutic intent with the patient's condition. If the diagnosis indicates a clear mechanical/structural condition, instrumental manipulation will be the most effective approach. If the diagnosis indicates a psychosomatic condition, expressive manipulation will be more suitable. This does not exclude the possibility that both forms of touch intent will be used simultaneously. For example, long-term stress may eventually lead to length changes in muscle. In this latter condition, instrumental manipulation will be used to stretch the muscle physically, while expressive manipulation will be used concomitantly to provide support and help the patient to relax.

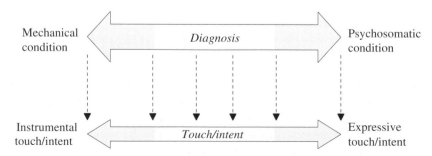

Figure 15.10   Relating the form of touch/intent to the patient's condition.

FORMS AND CONTENTS OF EXPRESSIVE TOUCH

Surprisingly little is written about expressive manipulation in manual therapy. There may be many reasons for this, one being the drive for acceptance and professionalism. Remen et al[81] have pointed out that 'human caring, sharing, feeling, accepting, touching and nourishing may all be thought of as manifestations of the feminine principle – the dimension which has been generally repressed in the modern view of professionalism'.

Martin Buber,[82] founder of the philosophy of encounter and dialogue, does not specifically refer to touch in his philosophy. However, Buber's concepts of relating can be very helpful in understanding the meaning of therapeutic touch. The basis of his philosophy lies in the concept of I–It and I–Thou. The I–It relating is object oriented. It reduces the other person to qualities or components, like the mechanical parts of a watch.[83] I–Thou relating perceives the other as a unified whole, with acceptance and mutuality. The other person is conceived as being as irreducible and autonomous as oneself. The I–It concept is very similar to the instrumental approach in manual therapy, in which the subject becomes an object – a mechanical entity. I–Thou relating is closer to the concept of expressive touch. Here the therapist is interacting with the patient as a whole person rather then just as a mechanical entity. The building blocks of such therapeutic interaction are individuality, personhood, inwardness of consciousness, sympathy, empathy and compassion. Although Buber sees I–It relating as a negative form of interaction between individuals, it must be emphasized that the instrumental part of a treatment is extremely important, as has been discussed in the previous two Sections: local repair processes in tissues can be affected by this form of manipulation.

To understand what constitutes expressive touch, one needs to look at therapeutic disciplines in which the use of expressive touch is well developed. One such unusual place is psychotherapy. Although in general psychotherapy touch is rarely used, even to the extent of not shaking the patient's hand, touch, in particular expressive touch, is commonly used in an area called 'body-psychotherapy'. Many of the models for body work in these disciplines are derived from the work of Wilhelm Reich, who developed a body-oriented approach to psychotherapy, in which touch and body contact play important therapeutic roles.[84] One such Neo-Reichian school is that of biodynamic psychotherapy, developed by Gerda Boyesen. Boyesen observed that her tactile contacts with the patients had a profound influence on their emotion and behaviour, and she thus extensively developed the use of touch as a psychotherapeutic tool. Bioenergetics and Gestalt,[47] all influenced by Reich, further developed the therapeutic use of touch. Manual methods used in these disciplines can give much insight into the contents and forms of expressive touch.[85]

For example, passive techniques are about letting go of control and trusting others, while active techniques are to do with trusting oneself and others (the therapist).[86] Active techniques can highlight strengths and weaknesses in relation to other individuals. Passive stretching can give a sense of openness of mind and a general sense of outflow, whilst active techniques can support a sense of containment. Deep work may give a feeling of being psychologically met; light work is less physically invasive (depending on the area being touched, its taboo value and its symbolism). Light touch could be used as a reminder, directing the patient's attention to specific areas of the body; static touch could imply contact and the therapist's presence.[47] Further to these examples, Figure 15.11 provides other elements which make up expressive touch.

It should be noted that these descriptions of expressive touch are very generalized and that expressive touch will change from one patient to another depending on a multitude of variables. How the patient responds to the different types of manipulation is also highly individualistic, so devising a standardized therapeutic approach is virtually impossible. The choice of techniques ultimately depends on feedback from the patient and the ability of the therapist to perceive and understand these messages.

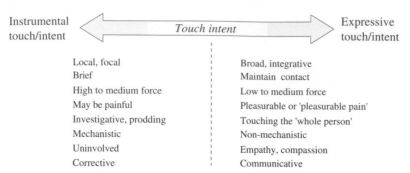

Figure 15.11 Some ingredients of instrumental and expressive manipulation. These ingredients lie within a spectrum of touch/intent, which depending on the patient's condition, may lean more in one direction or contain a complex mixture of these ingredients. Ideally, even highly instrumental treatments should contain some elements of expressive touch.

Touching the patient is not necessarily a communicative, expressive event: treatment can be highly mechanistic and emotionally detached even though touch is being used. Even when treatment is mechanistic, it is always advisable to include some elements of expressive touch. We do not treat machines but individuals like ourselves. If, for example, I manipulate a patient's knee, I always remind myself that there is a person 'behind the knee' and that I am also touching the whole person rather than just a mechanical hinge (which can sometimes be forgotten).

Developing instrumental touch relates to the therapist's improving his or her dexterity, motor coordination, manual skill and knowledge of anatomy and physiology. The development of expressive manipulation/touch is more complex and is related to the therapist's own maturity, personal growth, interpersonal and communication skills, and life experiences.

16

The psychosomatic sequence

When the patient is touched, the response is not only a 'mind' event, but also has physical bodily manifestations. These responses to manipulation are broad and non-specific physiological events that can be observed in several systems: as general changes in muscle tone, as altered autonomic and visceral activity, as altered pain perception and as the facilitation of healing and self-regulation. These psyche to soma responses are organized in an area of the brain called the limbic system.

THE LIMBIC SYSTEM

To understand the function of the limbic system, it is necessary to have a brief look at the overall anatomy of the nervous system. The nervous system is shaped like a mushroom (Fig. 16.1), the spinal cord and supraspinal centres forming its stem. The higher centres, such as the cortex, form

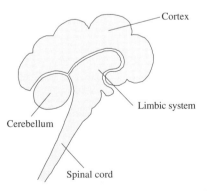

Figure 16.1   The brain is shaped like a mushroom. The limbic system is situated at the junction of the cap and stem, i.e. of the cortex, spinal and supraspinal centres.

the cap of the mushroom. In evolutionary terms, the stem is an early structure and is capable only of stereotyped and automated behaviour. The cap is a more recent structure and is associated with what makes humans more 'intelligent'.[87] The limbic area is situated between the stem and the cap. This makes it an important integration point between psychological and physiological processes.[88,89]

Function of the limbic system

The limbic system is where the muscular and visceral 'meets the emotional' or where 'emotion meets the soma'. The limbic area integrates emotional states such as anxiety, anger, depression, tension arousal, somnolent emotional states (relaxation) and states of emotional well-being.[88] It is an area of the brain in which the somatization of many psychological states take place and is involved in the control and expression of the individual's emotional behaviour and drives. The limbic system also organizes many of the body's physiological activities through its influence over the autonomic, neuroendocrine and motor systems. Physiological activities that are under the direct control of the limbic system are quite diverse: body temperature, osmolarity, body weight, the drive to eat and drink to name but a few (Fig. 16.2).[88] The integration of emotion

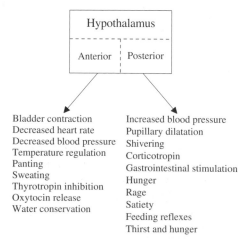

Figure 16.2 Some behavioural and somatic responses regulated by the hypothalamus, a part of the limbic system.

with physiology can be seen in, for example, the fright–flight–fight response, in which fear is somatized as a patterned protective response spanning the autonomic, neuroendocrine and motor systems. A similar protective response can be seen when electrical stimulation is directly applied to certain parts of the limbic system. In this situation, the animal will progress from being docile to showing aggressive behaviour, with all the related somatic/physiological responses.[90]

It should be noted that the perception of and response to manipulation are 'whole nervous system' events that are not restricted to the limbic system. Any given behaviour is controlled by extensive activity in various centres and networks of the nervous system. However, any function is usually dependent on one specific centre/area/network in the nervous system.[71] As such, the organization of the psychosomatic response is highly dependent on the limbic area.

THREE PATHWAYS TO PSYCHOSOMATIC EXPRESSION

In response to the needs, stimuli, drives and motivation of the individual, the limbic system organizes the physiological response, which is transmitted somatically via three routes (Fig. 16.3):

- the motor system
- the autonomic system
- the neuroendocrine system (via the pituitary gland).

The limbic system is capable of producing profound somatic responses, some of which are described below. Not all of these psychosomatic responses occur during a manual treatment, but they are included here to demonstrate the complexities, potency and patterns of the responses. This could help to explain some of the whole-person changes that may accompany a manual treatment.

MOTOR PATHWAY

Various emotional states can alter the general

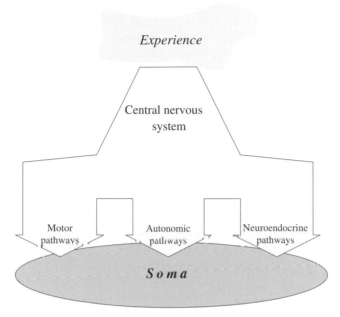

Experience

Central nervous system

Motor pathways

Autonomic pathways

Neuroendocrine pathways

S o m a

Figure 16.3   Three physiological pathways in the psychosomatic response.

motor tone throughout the body. Emotional states such as anxiety, anger, depression, tension and excitement are often accompanied by a generalized increase in muscle tone.[88,91,92] In contrast, somnolent emotional states (relaxation) and states of emotional well-being are usually associated with reduced overall muscular tone.[88] Each emotion is accompanied by a characteristic muscular response seen as alteration in posture and changes in facial expression.[92,93]

The limbic system, through the activity of the hypothalamus, can affect general motor tone. The anterior and posterior hypothalamus have a reciprocal relationship: when the activity of one area is increased, the activity of the other lessens. For example, when the activity in the anterior hypothalamus rises, there is a concomitant reciprocal inhibition of the posterior hypo-thalamus.[93] An increase in the activity of the anterior hypothalamus leads to increased sym-pathetic activity, motor discharges and cortical excitation.[94] An increase in the activity of the posterior hypothalamus leads to a parasym-pathetic response, with a reduction in motor tone.[95]

Response of the motor pathway to manipulation

General motor relaxation is often observed in manual treatments. This response is probably organized by the limbic system. In animal studies, it has been demonstrated that stroking the animal's back stimulates the anterior hypothalamic region, resulting in altered cortical activity, diminished gamma discharges and muscle relaxation.[94] There is some evidence that touch can produce such relaxation responses in non-conscious humans. There is a congenital anomaly in which infants are born without the cerebral hemispheres but with an intact lower part of the nervous system, such as the limbic areas (these infants are limbic in their behaviour). Many limbic functions are retained, such as crying in distress.[96] When the infant cries, stroking produces muscle relaxation and cessa-tion of crying.[93] This implies that the effects of stroking do not have to reach consciousness and that the response can be integrated in lower parts of the nervous system. It should be noted, however, that in this latter example these responses occur in the absence of influences from higher centres. The response may be different in a complete nervous system where the function of the limbic system is 'supervised' by the neocortex, which provides fine tuning of, and variety to the emotions.[89] Therefore, in a complete system, the individual's past experiences have a bearing on the activity of the limbic system. This could result in repression of the response of the person to being touched, without a change in general motor tone. The touch experience may also initiate a state of arousal and an increase in general motor tone (see below).

AUTONOMIC PATHWAY

The autonomic nervous system organizes the body's physiology for rapid responses. It comprises two pathways: the sympathetic and the parasympathetic. Generally speaking, the sympathetic system innervates larger parts of the body and therefore tends to have a more diffuse influence. It is associated with arousal states such as those brought on by stress and anxiety. The parasympathetic system is anatomically less diffuse and its effects are therefore more confined. It controls visceral activity or caretaker activities, and is associated with non-arousal states such as relaxation (Fig. 16.4).[93]

The effect of arousal or stress can be clearly seen in all autonomic responses, for example when subjects are asked to perform mental arithmetic. They will show many signs of the fright–flight–fight response: increase in systolic blood pressure, vasoconstriction in the superficial blood vessels and shunting of blood to skeletal muscles, thus increasing blood flow through the muscle by vasodilatation.[97] In such 'subtle' stressful situations, cardiovascular responses can be quite extensive: systolic blood pressure increases by 15%, heart rate by 33% and blood flow through (forearm) muscle by 334%. In some subjects, blood flow through muscle may increase by a staggering 773%.[96]

Response of the autonomic pathway to touch

Touching humans or animals is usually accompanied by an autonomic response. One method of observing this change is to record the activity of the cardiovascular system.[97] For example, when a dog is touched, there is a drop in its heart beat and blood pressure.[99] In extreme cases, this drop can be from 180 beats/min to 29 beats/min, accompanied by a 50% drop in systolic blood pressure. Similar changes have been observed in other animals, such as horses.[98]

A surprising finding is that when touch is applied to an unconscious and comatose person, similar changes occur in the cardiovascular system. In a study carried out at a shock trauma unit, it was shown that when the nurse held the patient's hands and quietly comforted him, heart rate would drop by as much as 30 beats/min.[100] The tactile sensations had 'filtered through' despite the fact that many of these patients had severe sensory bombardment from their injuries and medical interventions. It seems that the nervous system has a powerful capacity to recognize touch patterns even at such extreme conditions, and that this can happen in non-wakeful states or in unconsciousness. This is supported by the observation that encephalic babies who have no cortex will respond to human touch when in distress by ceasing to cry.

Another indication that manipulation can affect sympathetic activity via the limbic system comes from measuring the levels of body sweat before and after treatment. During arousal, there is an increase in body sweating related to increased sympathetic activity. It has been shown

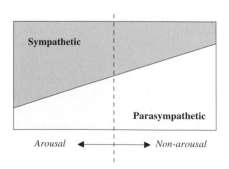

Figure 16.4 The role of the autonomic system in arousal and non-arousal states.

that when a subject receives a back massage, the sweating decreases, indicating a diminished sympathetic activity or reduced arousal.[107] Providing the manipulation is perceived as being positive by the patient, the overall effect is usually sedative and parasympathetic in nature. As has previously been stated (see also below) inappropriate touch may, however, result in an autonomic arousal state.

NEUROENDOCRINE PATHWAY

The neuroendocrine system plays a major role in self-regulation and affects virtually every process in the body. The hypothalamus plays a major role in integrating neuroendocrine activity. It releases a group of substances that stimulate the pituitary gland to secrete various hormones,[102] which act on different target endocrine systems in the body. For example, the hypothalamus secretes corticotropin-releasing factor, which in turn stimulates the pituitary to secrete the hormone ACTH. ACTH is released into the general circulation to stimulate its target, the adrenal gland, resulting in the synthesis and secretion of glucocorticoids, in particular hydrocortisone (an anti-inflammatory agent), adrenaline and noradrenaline (catecholamines). Adrenaline causes, for example, vasodilatation of blood vessels in skeletal muscle.

Psychological influences are one of the most potent activators of the hypothalamus–pituitary pathway.[103,104] Selye,[105] who developed the concept of the general stress syndrome, was able to show that the neuroendocrine system will respond to a wide range of psychological arousal states, such as fear, apprehension, anxiety, loud noises and crowding. There is a marked difference in the neuroendocrine response between individuals. Under stress, some subjects may demonstrate a continuous increase in their circulating hormonal levels, whilst others have the ability to adapt to long-term stress and may exhibit reduced or normal neuroendocrine activity. For example, studies of soldiers have demonstrated that some individuals are able to suppress their neuroendocrine activity on stressful days.[103,104]

Varying levels of arousal result in increased levels of synthesis and release of these hormones in the body. These responses have been demonstrated in 'benign' to 'severe' forms of stress. In the benign range are watching a violent film or performing a stressful mental task, such as mental arithmetic or sitting examinations.[106,107] In the severe range of stress lie experiences such as hospitalization, sleep deprivation, grief, anxiety and mental illness.[103,104] It is not only stressful events that activate the neuroendocrine system, but also pleasant emotional experiences such as watching something amusing or erotic.[108] Not surprisingly, watching a Disney nature film tends to reduce the level of arousal and the neuroendocrine response (could this be the antidote to executive stress?).[109]

Prolonged arousal and stress is associated with a related long-term increase in the hormonal levels, which is believed to account for various illnesses. For example, the effect of the stress of modern living has been shown to affect the cardiovascular system by causing an increase in the levels of circulating catecholamines. These are believed to be the cause of degenerative cardiovascular disease.[89] In healthy animals, such cardiovascular lesions can be produced by stress brought about by a prolonged alteration in social and behavioural habits.[110] Similar pathological mechanisms may underlie the occurrence of death following prolonged grief periods. It has been reported that, in widowers, there is an increased mortality rate within the first 6 months after the loss of their partner.[110] Similarly, prolonged psychiatric illness and neurosis can reduce life expectancy.[89] In long-term depression, there are signs of abnormal endocrine activity (initiated by the hypothalamus), resulting in hypersecretion of hormones such as cortisone or reduced levels of growth hormone.[111] Such long-term alterations in hormonal levels are probably the cause of the growth failure seen in socially deprived children.

The potent relationship between emotion and somatic responses can be seen on rare occasions in otherwise healthy individuals. Even short periods of extreme stress can lead to illness and death. Sudden death of otherwise normal individuals can happen within hours or days of a shocking experience, as has been documented in voodoo rituals in which the medicine man makes a death suggestion towards the victim.[112] The victim, usually male, dies within 24 hours from severe emotional shock. Similar sudden death of healthy individuals was recorded during the London air raids of World War II. Sudden death can be induced in experimental animals by exposure to high levels of stress. This severe response is probably limbic in origin and is mediated via the autonomic and neuroendocrine systems.

Circulating hormones have also been shown to affect the brain's pattern of electrical activity and therefore an individual's behaviour. This can result in convulsion and may also affect a person's behavioural development.[105] There is evidence that many of these hormonal responses can be normalized once the level of arousal is reduced.[104] For example, during stress and anxiety, the flow through skeletal muscles rises as a result of raised levels of circulating adrenaline and increased sympathetic activity.[112] Decreasing the patient's anxiety level can normalize the vasodilatation, indicating a more balanced physiological activity. In psychiatric patients who have unusually high catecholamine levels, a positive improvement in their condition is associated with a lowering of these levels.[104] It has also been demonstrated that, during a hypnotic trance, which is associated with deep relaxation, neuroendocrine activity tends to be reduced.[114]

Effects of manipulation on neuroendocrine activity

Long-term responses to manual therapy probably relate to its influences upon the neuroendocrine system. In young animals, tactile contacts have been shown to have wide physiological effects through activation of the neuroendocrine system, thus influencing many cellular processes in the body. These effects have been observed in animal brain, liver, heart, kidney, lung and spleen.[9] Similar neuroendocrine responses to tactile stimulation are seen in human infants. These effects have been extensively discussed at the beginning of this section. Whether human touch has similar effects on adults is at present unknown. In my own practice, I have on numerous occasions seen changes in the physical and psychological state of the patient that cannot be explained by a biomechanical model but can only be attributed to the effect of manipulation on the limbic and neuroendocrine systems.

MANIPULATION: RELAXATION OR AROUSAL?

As has previously been discussed, some studies demonstrate that touch or massage may reduce arousal, implicating reduced sympathetic activity. However, manipulation may provoke the opposite effect: an increase in arousal, and sympathetic activity. For example, back massage has been shown to cause a general increase in sympathetic activity, manifested as a slight increase in heart and breathing rate.[115] Although this study had its flaws, it does point to an important principle: that manipulation can either be stimulating, resulting in an arousal state, or, in different circumstances, promote non-arousal and relaxation. There are several variables that will determine the direction of response:

1. The manual event itself may have sedative or stimulating elements. A vigorous massage, articulation, high-velocity thrusts (adjustments), strong and deep treatment could all initiate an arousal response. This may be related to the patient perceiving the manipulation as being aggressive, something to protect oneself against by tensing up (which may be exacerbated if the treatment inflicts pain). In contrast, gentle massage, holding techniques and gentle body rocking will generally reduce arousal and promote relaxation.

2. The therapist's intention: a comforting and supportive manipulation may help to reduce arousal and promote relaxation. In contrast, if the therapist communicates a sexual or aggressive tactile message, the patient may feel uneasy or threatened, which may result in increased arousal.

3. The patient's interpretation of touch (Fig. 16.5). This relates to patients' previous experiences of touch within the whole psychosocial context of their life. Therefore, the way in which the patient may perceive touch can be very complex. In general, if the patient has no aversion to touch, it is likely that he or she will perceive manipulation as a positive experience, with reduced arousal. If the patient has had a negative tactile experience, such as physical abuse, another person's touch may be a source of

fear and arousal, no matter how positive the therapist's intentions may be.

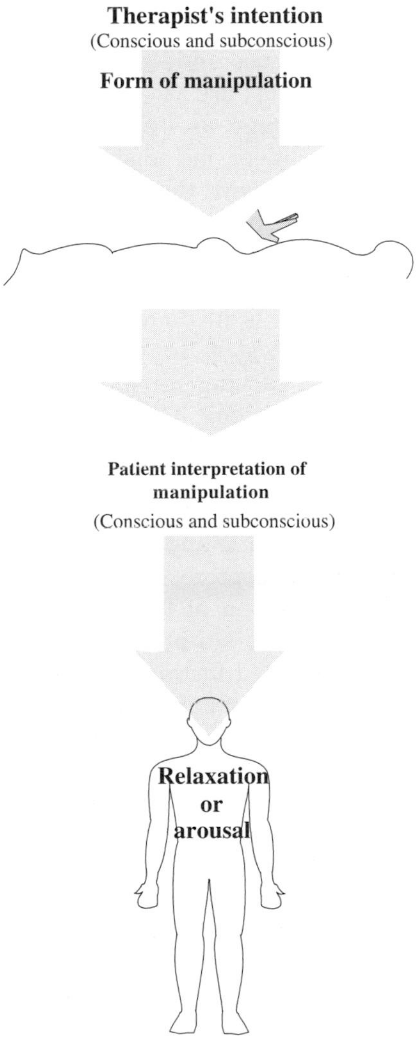

PSYCHOSOMATIC VERSUS SOMATOVISCERAL REFLEXES

The principle that manipulation is able reflexly to alter autonomic activity is found in several manual therapies. One commonly held belief is that stimulation of proprioceptors will affect visceral activity via a spinal reflex mechanism. This reflex pathway is called the somatovisceral reflex. The concept of the somatovisceral reflex proposes that the proprioceptive stimulus does not need to reach the higher brain centres but occurs within sympathetic centres in the spinal cord. In this reflex arc, the stimulation of proprioceptors in one segmental area will affect the related segmental autonomics and viscera. According to this principle, if the upper thoracic area is manipulated by high-velocity thrust or massage, it may help to regulate the autonomic activity to the heart. Similarly, if the lower part of the thoracic spine is manipulated, it may affect gut activity. Thus, the reflex response is organ specific, related to the particular segmental spinal autonomics. Counter to the somatovisceral reflex stands the processes discussed in this section: manipulation as having a potent effect on psychosomatic processes. This is a non-specific, generalized response that is not related to a single or a group of spinal segments, and is organized by higher brain centres such as the limbic system.

There are many flaws in the somatovisceral model, some of which are noted below:

Firstly, in the intact animal, the centres above the spinal cord have a dominant role in controlling and regulating autonomic activity, and spinal centres are under the direct influence of these centres.[116,118,119]

Second, somatovisceral reflexes have been demonstrated in several studies.[116,120] However, in all studies, the animal has to have severe autonomic disability before the responses can be shown. The studies usually involve the sectioning of various higher autonomic centres (situated above the spinal cord).[116-119] Under

Figure 16.5 Depending on different variables, a manual event can result in either relaxation or arousal.

these experimental conditions, some changes in gut or cardiovascular activity may be observed by stimulating different proprioceptors.[118,119] Similar responses can be seen in trauma patients whose spinal cord has been severed and 'disconnected' from the higher centres.[121] In these individuals, mass reflexes can be observed, in which the stimulation of proprioceptors can provoke an autonomic–visceral response. However, if some parts of the higher centres are left intact, they tend to override the somatovisceral reflexes.[122] The response of spinal autonomics to proprioceptive stimulation in the spinal animal is probably related to the 'law of denervation' which states that the elimination of normal central influences on neurons may sensitize them to other stimulating factors.[123] Furthermore, in many of these studies, stimulation consists of a large electric shock to the receptor's fibre rather than stimulating the receptor itself. These extreme conditions never occur in real-life situations and cannot therefore be expected to occur during manipulation.[124]

Third, in the somatosympathetic concept, the spinal segments are usually described as being anatomically discrete, although it is doubtful whether such anatomical specificity occurs within the spinal cord. As has been discussed in Section 2, proprioceptors are not segment specific, and their fibres tend to ascend and descend in the spinal cord over a few segments. Similarly, motorneurons lack any segmental specificity. They are intermingled within the ventral horn column of the spinal cord. It is to be expected that autonomic motor centres are just as integrated within the cord. The confusion arises because afferent and efferent fibres are anatomically distinct when they enter and exit the intervertebral foramina. Once in the spinal cord, this anatomical order is lost. Indeed, when proprioceptors are stimulated, there is a mass sympathetic excitation rather than a specific segmental response.[116] If the somatic afferents of the hindlimb or forelimb of a spinal animal are stimulated, the sympathetic response tends to be similar, i.e. irrespective of the anatomical specificity of the proprioceptors.

Fourth, reflexive control over the autonomic

nervous system has no biological logic. If proprioceptors had autonomic control, it would mean that movement or peripheral damage would influence visceral activity. An injury occurring in a particular dermatome would affect the visceral activity associated with that segment, a broken rib, for example, because of its segmental connection, causing cardiac changes. Along the same lines, if a vertebra were crushed or a disc herniated, one would expect visceral changes associated with the damaged segment. Such events could never happen in real life as they would defy survival principles: not only would the animal be injured, but it would now also have to deal with the internal visceral mayhem that such an injury would cause. Indeed, disc injuries and crushed vertebra that are associated with severe proprioceptive change, as well as an increase in sensory bombardment, fail to show any visceral changes associated with the damaged segment. This is supported by clinical observation that musculoskeletal injuries are rarely if ever accompanied by visceral changes. The only visceral response to injury is mediated centrally, probably by the limbic system, for example, following a severe injury, causing an individual to feel nauseous. The autonomic nervous system is well protected against somatovisceral reflexes from proprioceptors.

The only exception to the above is the sympathetic supply to muscle and skin, which may be affected by proprioceptors. This is related to the sympathetic regulation of local activity such as blood flow and perspiration, which has an important regulatory function with respect to the cellular environment of the tissues. However, it is unclear what role manual therapy can play in such complex regulation.

Fifth, Sherrington has predicted that proprioceptors are exclusively part of the motor system.[125] As discussed in Section 2, they provide feedback rather than control the motor system. It would be expected that, in the intact animal, they would have an even smaller influence over spinal autonomic centres, or even none at all.

The autonomic nervous system has its own mechanoreceptors: baroreceptors, enteric receptors and other non-mechanical receptors such as chemoreceptors.[126,127] Gut activity is controlled by the enteric nervous system (under the influence of higher autonomic centres), which has its own specialized group of mechanoreceptors embedded within the gut wall. It is an almost autonomous system within the autonomic nervous system, controlling such events as gut peristalsis. It is very unlikely that this system would be reflexively affected by musculoskeletal mechanoreceptors.

Sixth, if the somatovisceral concept is accepted, the question arises of how to sustain the changes brought about by manipulation. Could a single thrust of a dorsal facet joint alter cardiovascular pathology? Could it alter the gut motility of a person suffering from irritable bowel syndrome or peptic ulcer? I believe that the answer to these questions is no. If it were possible to affect visceral activity, repetition of the manual event would have to be extensive, outside the limits of clinical feasibility.

Last, in all of the above-cited studies, stimulation of proprioceptors results in *excitation* of the sympathetic nervous system. If it were possible to affect this system by manipulation, it would result in *excitation*, rather than inhibition,

of some organs, for example the cardiovascular system. To effectively reduce cardiac activity, the parasympathetic system has to be stimulated (or sympathetic activity somehow reduced). Parasympathetic activity is regulated by higher centres in the nervous system rather than by spinal centres, giving a generalized rather than a segmental response. To complicate the issue further, parasympathetic input will reduce cardiac activity but increase the secretomotor activity of the gut. How these fine variables can be controlled by manipulation have never been addressed. One needs to consider such important questions as, how does one know when manipulation is inhibitory or excitatory to either the sympathetic or parasympathetic system?

Our conclusion falls in line with the summary of Section 2. Basically, an individual cannot be regarded as a set of reflexes that can be manipulated from the periphery. Many of the autonomic responses seen following manipulation are probably related to autonomic descending influences from higher brain centres (Fig. 16.6). In order specifically to affect visceral activity, it is more likely that direct manipulation such as vis-

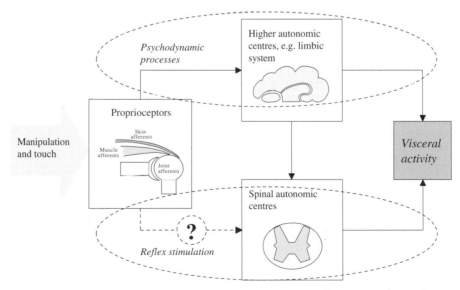

Figure 16.6 The effect of manipulation on visceral activity is unlikely to occur via reflex stimulation of spinal autonomic centres. Most manual influences are related to the psychodynamics of touch and its effect on the limbic system.

ceral techniques will be more effective. However, there is to date little research in manual therapy to support the use of visceral manipulation.

PSYCHOSOMATIC TEMPLATES

Every emotion is associated with a patterned somatic response or at least with an impulse towards it – a somatic pattern displaying the individual's state of mind.[51] Many somatic responses have a biological meaning and are related to physiological and musculoskeletal support for the expression of the emotions.[89] Behaviour occurs in fairly patterned responses involving motor, autonomic and neuroendocrine activity.[52,128,129] These stereotyped responses will be termed *psychosomatic templates* (Fig. 16.7). These 'preprogrammed' patterns can be seen in emotions such as happiness, sadness, anger and fear. Darwin,[128] who is usually associated with evolution rather than emotion, made an extensive study of emotions and their somatic expression. He writes that the most common and basic expressive actions exhibited by man and the lower animals are innate, genetic or inherited. Most reactions are neither learned nor imitated, and are beyond our control. Darwin gives the examples of vascular changes in the skin in blushing, and the increased action of the heart in

anger. His overall conclusion is 'that the young and the old of widely different races, both with man and animals, express the same state of mind by the same movements.'

Some elements of the response, such as changes in facial expression and whole-body posture (the musculoskeletal part of the template), are visually apparent. Some of the autonomic changes, for example blushing, blanching and perspiring, or changes in the depth and rate of breathing, are also 'overt'.[89,130] These are the external manifestation of the templates, but 'covert' internal changes also take place. For example, it is known that the lining of the stomach reacts to emotions such as pleasure, fear, anger and pain.[130] Recruitment of other body systems in the expression of emotion has been discussed above.

PSYCHOSOMATIC TEMPLATES IN PSYCHOSOMATIC ILLNESS

Emotional life is a continuum from one emotional state to another. A state of depression may be followed by any number of possible emotional combinations – happiness followed by grief, followed by anxiety – each with its different duration and intensity. On such an emotional rollercoaster, the somatic responses follow suit, with movements from one somatic state to

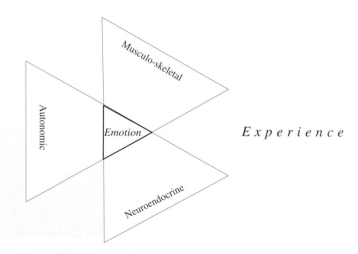

Figure 16.7 The psychosomatic template has three physiological limbs.

another (Fig. 16.8). If the system is healthy and has a functional flexibility, it will freely move from one state to another without any residual problem. In health, the somatic responses are transient and last as long as the emotion that lies at their root. Psychosomatic illness may arise when the person is 'stuck' or has recurrent episodes in one pattern of emotion over a long period of time, for example when under chronic emotional stress and anxiety. In these circumstances, a continuous somatic response is maintained and may, in the long term, have pathological effects on normal motor and autonomic function, such as an increase in blood pressure, an increase in the secretion of digestive acids, or increased muscle tension in the shoulders. The effects of chronic stress are well documented. In unemployed men, who are expected to be under stress, blood pressure was found to be higher throughout the unemployment period, returning to normal when work was resumed.[89] Similarly, pulse rate in chronically stressed individuals tends to be higher than in normal people, in both stress and

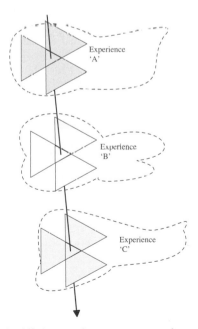

Figure 16.8 Life is a continuous movement from one emotion to another. The three psychosomatic pathways recruit parts of the body in different somatic patterns to follow these changes.

rest conditions.[131] In the long term, these continuous physiological assaults could initiate a pathological process in the end-organ or tissue. For example, an increase in blood pressure can affect the brain, heart, kidneys and blood vessel walls.[89,132,133] A rise in the secretion of digestive fluid may promote the formation of ulcers,[133] and an increase in muscle tone may lead to musculoskeletal pain and pathology.

Although the psychosomatic response is fairly patterned, individual differences can be seen in the magnitude of the response of a particular body system rather than in a change of pattern.[129] This difference in magnitude can be clearly observed in the expression of anger. One individual will shake his fists, whilst another may just clench them. Similarly, during stress, heart and blood pressure tend to rise. However, the individual variation or amplitude of response can be quite wide.

The question arises of how a normal psychosomatic response turns into a pathological process. This seems to be related to the two ends of the psychosomatic response. At one end is the magnitude and duration of the emotional state,[132] at the other, the physiological integrity or vulnerability of the end-organ or system.[132] Problems may arise when the individual is subjected to extreme or chronic emotional stress as this will lead to overloading of the end-organs or systems (Fig. 16.9). If the organ or system is 'healthy', it will probably adapt well to this severe demand. If, however, there are areas of vulnerability in the body, severe acute or chronic stress may exhaust the weaker organ or system, leading to its failure.[135] It should be noted that psychosomatic illness does not always develop as a result of a major life crisis but can develop from the frequent hassles of daily living.[136]

Vulnerability of an organ or a system can result from different aetiologies, such as genetic, or acquired from illness, operation or injuries that are not psychosomatic in origin.[130,132] It is also possible to acquire a pattern of response by a learning process (similar to conditioning), which will increase the demand on an organ or system during times of arousal.[137] In my practice, I often see psychosomatic symptoms that manifest

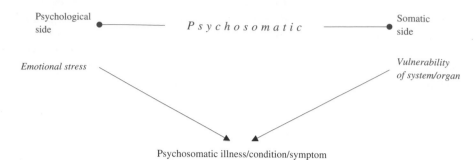

Figure 16.9 Possible mechanisms in the development of a psychosomatic illness/condition/symptom.

themselves in weak areas of the body, such as old musculoskeletal injuries or areas of past surgery. The most simple example is shoulder and neck tension in stress. Although virtually every individual has a stereotypic response of tensing the shoulders in response to stress, not all will suffer from neck problems. It is assumed that those with postural problems, wear and tear problems or past whiplash injuries will suffer most as this becomes a source of weakness. If we take as an example the study quoted above on unemployed men displaying increased blood pressure, we can see a group of individuals sharing a common experience with a fairly similar pattern of autonomic activity, i.e. increased blood pressure. However, only a small number, probably those with a vulnerable cardiovascular system, will develop cardiovascular pathology.

PSYCHOSOMATIC CONDITIONS AS AN ADAPTIVE RESPONSE

Some psychosomatic illnesses may be related to an individual's tendency subconsciously (or less commonly consciously) to augment particular pathways or physiological responses in certain areas of the body. The organ or system under focus may be physiologically normal to begin with, but with heightened stimulation may eventually fail (Fig. 16.10). For example, a child may 'learn' to control parts of his autonomic nervous system in order to seek attention or avoid an unpleasant and stressful event such as going to school.[135] He may find that, by turning pale or vomiting, he will be allowed to stay at

home. With repetition, this becomes a patterned response, which may in adult life accompany situations of anxiety or stress. In these circumstances, emotions of fear and anxiety will then tend to be magnified around the gut and may result in malfunction of that area.

Many of these mind – body relationships arise from psychological and somatic protective and adjustive patterns developed for survival in a hostile or negative environment. These patterns are usually connected with conflicts or the withholding of expression.[138] Reich[139] termed these patterns of tension 'body armouring'. They can arise from sudden shock, anxiety or conflicts of emotional interests where full expression is not permitted so is repressed. For every emotion,

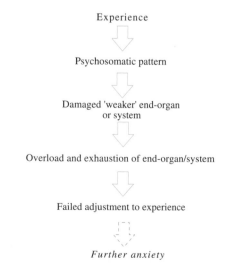

Figure 16.10 A possible mechanism of psychosomatic illness.

there is a psychological and somatic cycle, a continuous movement from tension to release.[46] However, if the cycle is not allowed to run to completion, it will manifest itself in a psychological and somatic armouring. In Reich's words: 'Every increase of muscular tonus and rigidification is an indication that a vegetative excitation, anxiety, or sexual sensation has been blocked and bound'.[139] Stewart & Joines[140] write, 'It seems that we make some of our earliest decisions with our body as well as our minds. Perhaps the infant wants to reach out for mother. But he discovers that Mother often draws away from him. To quell the pain of this rejection, he suppresses his bodily urge. To stop himself reaching out, he tenses his arms and shoulders. Many years later as a grown-up, he may still hold this tension. But he will be unaware he is doing so. He may experience aches and pains in his shoulders or his neck'. They also add an important point for manual therapists. 'Under deep massage or in therapy, he may feel the tension and then release it. With that release, he is likely to release also the flood of feeling he had repressed since infancy.' These patterns of holding and not expressing may become entrenched, to form a stereotypic response throughout life – a psychosomatic template (Fig. 16.11). These patterns do not necessarily arise in childhood but can be acquired throughout life as a result of different experiences.

Further to the adaptive concept as a source of psychosomatic illness, there is also a symbolic model for psychosomatic illness.[117,134] As has been previously discussed, different areas, organs or systems of the body may have symbolic significance for the individual. Psychosomatic illness arises when the individual

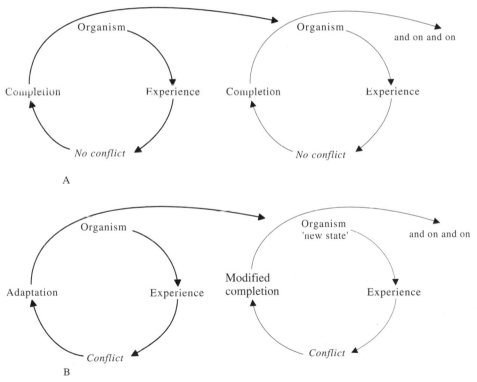

Figure 16.11 Behaviour as an adaptive process. (A) Each experience has a psychosomatic response that is cyclical in nature. When there is no conflict between behaviour and experience, the cycle is completed. (B) If conflict arises between experience and behaviour, an adjustment has to take place. This adaptation or new state could form the template for responses to subsequent experiences.

subconsciously uses that part of the body to express an emotion or make a statement.[141] The individual subconsciously 'disorganizes' or stresses the symbolic area, which may culminate in a pathological process. This may be seen in particular areas, organs or systems of the body, for example as musculoskeletal (e.g. low back pain), respiratory (e.g. asthma), digestive (e.g. peptic ulcers) or cardiovascular reactions (e.g. palpitations).

What is important to understand is that the human experience contains a variety of emotions, some of which we may perceive as 'negative' or 'positive' in nature. There is nothing biologically wrong in a negative emotion, with its physiological arousal: it is an adaptive process to ensure the survival of the individual.[142] The problem arises only when an emotion, usually a negative one, becomes unresolved and psychosomatically sustained, or so acute that it completely 'throws the body off'.

MANUAL THERAPY IN PSYCHOSOMATIC CONDITIONS

In practice, we often see patients whose psychosomatic symptoms or conditions resolve following manual treatment. If we are not providing psychotherapy, by what mechanism do they get better? How do these changes come about?

The psychosomatic response can be seen to start as an emotion expressed as behaviour and is ultimately dependent on the ability of the end-organ to support that behaviour. Different manual approaches can be addressed to each point in this sequence. At the emotional end of the sequence, manual therapy can take a supportive form, in the behavioural part, it can be in the form of behavioural therapy; and at the end-organ stage, it can occur as physical therapy. Thus manipulation may have multiple roles in treating psychosomatic conditions (Fig. 16.12):

- manipulation as supportive therapy
- manipulation as behavioural therapy
- manipulation as physical therapy.

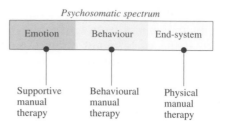

Figure 16.12 The possible role of manual therapy in treating psychosomatic conditions.

MANIPULATION AS SUPPORTIVE THERAPY

The supportive role of manual therapy can be often seen in the treatment of psychosomatic conditions. Patients frequently present with physical symptoms but no history of injury or pathology. The onset of symptoms can often be traced to a period of emotional stress. The patient may describe back pain that started, for example, on becoming unemployed or losing a close relative. This change in symptomatic picture can occur even if the life situation has remained the same. Although some patients will need counselling, this is not always necessary for a positive outcome: manual treatment can be in itself psychologically supportive.

Touch that conveys non-verbal messages of comfort and support may help the patient during periods of heightened anxiety or stress by reducing the general level of arousal and bringing the body closer to the self-regulation levels present in non-stressful states (Fig. 16.13). Treatment could help to reduce the physiological overload on different body systems, including those weakened and vulnerable. For example, massage or other forms of manipulation may help to reduce the state of arousal in a patient with mild cardiovascular symptoms. This could lead to a reduction in the physiological loading of the cardiovascular system and subsequently to an improvement in symptoms. However, the generalized relaxation response is not organ or system specific but has a blanket effect: every organ and system is affected.

Reducing arousal may also help to conserve energy in the body and lessen the eventuality

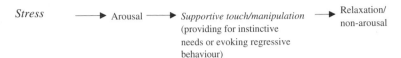

Stress ⟶ Arousal ⟶ *Supportive touch/manipulation* ⟶ Relaxation/
(providing for instinctive   non-arousal
needs or evoking regressive
behaviour)

Figure 16.13 Manipulation as supportive therapy.

of exhaustion in the different organs and systems. This principle can be demonstrated in the musculoskeletal system. During emotional tension there is a general increase in muscle tone, and the total metabolic activity of skeletal muscles and their energy consumption are greatly increased during emotional excitation. However, if the activity is carried out without emotional excitement, the metabolic activity tends to reduce, implying energy conservation.[93,143] This could be important to individuals who are under stress and complain of low energy and fatigue in their daily activities. It may also help explain generalized muscle pain that originates from fatigue in prolonged emotional states.

The supportive form of manual therapy probably accounts for many of the general somatic or physiological changes and the consequent improvement in the patient's psychosomatic symptomatology. This by no means aims to imply that manual therapy should replace psychotherapy in treating psychosomatic conditions. However, it does imply that some psychosomatic conditions will (and do) respond to manual therapy without the use of psychotherapy.

MANIPULATION AS BEHAVIOURAL THERAPY

Manual guidance is another possible mechanism that could promote a change in the psychosomatic response. The therapist can raise awareness and guide the patient in reducing activity within one of the psychosomatic pathways. In this approach, the aim of treatment is to modify the psychosomatic template during situations of stress, for example, guiding a patient who suffers from neck tension in how to reduce motor activity and relax the neck at such times (Table 16.1). Eventually, and with adequate repetition, this will become a new, less exhausting psychosomatic pattern. (This form of treatment has been discussed in Section 2.)

The ability to induce a behavioural change relies on the notion that psychosomatic templates are not hard-wired but have a potential for neuroplasticity (see Section 2). There is much experimental evidence to suggest that the limbic system is plastic,[143] implying that the psychosomatic templates will adapt to new experiences. The most obvious evidence for this is that, throughout life, psychosomatic symptoms can change, indicating that new patterns can be acquired. Studies also demonstrate the ability of individuals to reduce, in the long term, the activity of one of the three psychosomatic pathways. This, too, may indicate a learning process and adaptation. For example, when using biofeedback methods, subjects suffering from irritable bowel syndrome showed a long-term improvement in their condition.[145,146] In these studies, a stethoscope was placed on the abdomen and the subject learnt mentally to manipulate the peristaltic sounds. The ability to reduce the sounds indicated a reduction in activity in the autonomic pathway. Using biofeedback, it has also been demonstrated that subjects can learn to control their heart rate:[147] subjects placed in a stressful situation can maintain their heart rate at a lower level. Control over the body's smooth muscle activity including the internal gut sphincters, is part of the Paula method (developed in Israel). In this method, the trainees learn, first by concentrating on external sphincter muscles (such as around the mouth, genitalia or eyes), to control deeper autonomically activated sphincters. Although the Paula method has no research to support it, claims for

Table 16.1 Muscular tension of the shoulders and neck as an example of different treatment approaches

	Supportive approach	Behavioural approach	Physical approach
Treatment aims	Reduce general arousal, leading to reduced demand on the musculoskeletal system	Promote change in the psychosomatic template Guide patient in how to reduce neck and shoulder tension during periods of stress	Improve function, promote change in structure of end-system/organ This may help end-system to cope better or adapt with more flexibility to periods of increased demand
Treatment	General non-specific relaxing manipulation	Hands of practitioner placed over tense muscle to gauge muscle tightness Patient is guided verbally as to level of muscle relaxation (manual feedback)	Reduce muscle shortening by stretch or soft-tissue massage to neck and shoulder muscles Active technique may help to promote neuromuscular adaptions and change Active techniques may also help to promote change in vascular supply to the muscles

the ability to control internal sphincters comes from a completely different source: sword-swallowers. According to the account of one sword-swallower, it takes about 2 years to learn to insert a sword into the throat while relaxing the oesophageal muscles.[135] From my own experience, in my high days of yoga, one of the internal cleansing methods was to try to swallow a 5 m length of gauze and then pull it out of the mouth. It took several months before I could learn to control my oesophagus, and even then I was only able to swallow about 1 m of cloth.

Pathway flexibility for adaptation

The ease with which the three pathways can be made to re-adapt depends on the extent to which they can be influenced by conscious processes. The neuromuscular pathway is probably the most adaptable of the three pathways as it can be controlled by volitional, conscious processes. It is also a highly adaptive system, which can, throughout life, learn new patterns of motor activity. In comparison, many visceral activities are automatic, non-conscious processes that can be controlled to some extent, but with more difficulty, by conscious cues and require longer guidance and feedback periods. One must remember that feedback is a way of bringing an automatic process into awareness. Musculoskeletal activity, being very 'close' to awareness, is much more approachable than is that of visceral systems, which are remote from consciousness.

Changes in autonomic patterns cannot be effectively produced without accurate and immediate feedback from the body. Within the constraints of manual therapy, there is no direct and reliable feedback from the organ or system. However, 'semiconscious' autonomic systems such as breathing may be open to manual feedback. To promote autonomic plasticity, other forms of biofeedback are probably more effective than manual therapy. This does not exclude the possible use of manual therapy in conjunction with biofeedback instrumentation; this, however, is outside the scope of this book.

MANIPULATION AS PHYSICAL THERAPY

Manual therapy as a physical therapy has been extensively described in Section 1, particularly in relation to the musculoskeletal system. Section 1 describes how the function and structure of end-organs, tissues or systems can be directly affected by manual therapy. From the psychosomatic perspective, an improvement in the end-organ would allow these structures to function more efficiently under stress and make them less likely to fail. The most accessible to manipulation of the body systems is, naturally enough, the musculoskeletal system. The relationship between improving the state of the end-tissue and its response to stress can be observed in many musculoskeletal injuries. For example, in whiplash injuries, it is very common to see an exaggeration of symptoms in the neck when the patient is under stress (Table 16.1). A manual treatment that improves cervical function and helps to reverse some of the structural damage will provide a better baseline for that area during periods of increased activity (such as stress).

In comparison to the musculoskeletal system, the visceral system is much less accessible to direct manipulation, although it is not impossible to reach most internal organs by direct deep manual pressure. It is, however, very doubtful whether manipulation can be used directly to influence internal organs to improve their function.

MANUAL BODY ROCKING

Body rocking and rhythmic techniques are used extensively in manual therapy. Procedures such as the harmonic technique[148] in osteopathy, the Traiger method and pulsing specialize in applying low-frequency mechanical vibration to the whole body or to the different body masses.

Therapeutic body rocking

The therapeutic origins of these techniques can be traced to intrauterine life and infancy. Whole-body rocking is a common form of deep proprioceptive stimulation used to calm babies. It is initiated either by the parent cradling and gently swinging the baby, or by having the baby strapped in a sling close to the body. As the parent moves, the baby is rocked in a complex pattern of movement.[148] Studies into the effect of whole-body rocking have demonstrated its potency in the young. When rocking was applied to newly born babies, it either delayed the onset of crying,[149] or stopped it.[6] This was found

to be more effective in reducing the infant's crying compared with verbal calming,[6] or touch alone.[150]

A rocking frequency of between 50 and 70 cycles per minute will invariably stop the baby crying. However, if the speed of rocking moves outside these levels, it does not seem to affect the baby's crying. Pulse rate measurements taken during rocking show a sharp decline to near resting level when the right frequency of rocking is reached. This cardiovascular effect is more marked than when the baby is given a dummy: with the dummy, the heart rate will drop, but it still does not reach the level achieved by rocking.[6]

The effects of rocking are not exclusive to humans. Harlow, in his studies of the attachment of infant monkeys to surrogate mothers, has also demonstrated that when the infant had the choice between a stationary and a rocking cloth mother, it invariably preferred the rocking mother.

One therapeutic use of body rocking is in treating disabled or hyperactive children. Ayers[151] states that vestibular stimulation is one of the most powerful tools available for therapeutic use in remedying problems of sensory integration and dysfunction in disabled children. This type of stimulation is achieved by passively rocking the child on a net hammock or by vibrating different parts of the body. In hyperactive children, such stimulation has been shown to reduce their excitatory state and general muscle tone.[151]

Another area in which whole-body rocking is used is in promoting the development of premature babies. Rocking and tactile stimulation have been shown to improve the infant's health in several areas. Preterm babies who received such stimulation were shown to catch up or even exceed the development of normal, full-term babies.[152] This can be in terms of improved weight gain, frequency of stools, reduced frequency of apnoea, reduced frequency of bradycardia (slowing of heart beat),[153] smoother and less jerky movements, and more spontaneous and mature motor behaviour with fewer signs of irritability and hypertonicity.[154–156]

Physiological mechanisms in body rocking

The mechanisms that underlie the changes seen in body rocking are associated with the stimulation of two sensory systems: the vestibular apparatus in the semicircular canals of the ear,[122] and proprioception from skin, joints and muscle receptors. This sensory flow, along with sensory information from vision and hearing, is processed in an area of the brain called the vestibular nucleus (Ch. 8).[152] The vestibular nucleus also organizes impulses from the brain stem, cerebellum and many parts of the cerebral cortex. A continuous flow of impulses from the vestibular nucleus plays a part in the generation of motor tone in postural muscles. Inhibition of this flow usually results in muscle relaxation, and excitation, in contration. Inhibition may occur in part through the vestibular nuclei activating the cerebellum, which in turn inhibits the brain stem reticular formation. It has been suggested that slow rhythmic rocking has an overall inhibitory influence by activating these pathways.[152] It should be noted that, although the rocking movements stimulate the vestibular apparatus, the overall relaxation response may also be attributed to the concurrent stimulation of skin receptors and the psychodynamic processes associated with it.[61]

These studies demonstrate the importance of movement and rhythm on psychosomatic processes, and that a relaxation response can occur during rhythmic/dynamic treatments rather than just during static manipulations. A patient who receives a rocking treatment will frequently describe their relaxation as very deep, almost trance-like. The nature of these techniques and their influence on the patient's mind prompted one student to describe body rocking as 'soft-tissue hypnosis'.

PAIN RELIEF BY MANIPULATION: PSYCHOLOGICAL PROCESSES

The role of manipulation in pain relief may be related to its being partly a regressive process. Just as the parent's touch is capable of calming a child who is in pain, so may the practitioner's touch induce a regressive state associated with the safety and comfort of early life. This could in return reduce the immediate state of stress and anxiety, resulting in higher tolerance to pain. It has been shown that the perception of pain is highly dependent on the patient's psychological state, anxiety, depression, low self-esteem, hysteria and anger all having been shown to reduce the tolerance of pain.[66,157] Korr[158] when describing the facilitated spinal segment, observed that emotional factors play an important role in the state of facilitation. Subjects who were apprehensive, anxious or emotionally upset often showed increased facilitation and a reduced pain threshold. Improvement in the different psychological states, for example anxiety and depression, is associated with an increased tolerance of pain.[66]

The physiological mechanism of pain reduction in manipulation is believed to be related to the potent inhibitory influences that the higher brain centres have on incoming pain sensations.[159] However, because these responses are psychological in origin, a central inhibition of pain may not be a stereotypic response in every patient. The potency of the response is related to various psychological factors as well as the patient–therapist relationship.

Pain relief observed during and following manipulation may be brought about by descending influences from higher brain centres. A large proportion of ascending fibres from the central nervous system have a strong influence over incoming sensory information at the spinal cord level (Fig. 16.14).[160] For example, direct stimulation of the sensorimotor area of the cortex or subcortical structures can exert a powerful inhibition on sensory activity at spinal level.[161–163] Long-term pain relief by stimulation of subcortical areas has been demonstrated in patients with chronic pain.[164] The long-term pain relief often seen following manipulation may be related to the effect that higher brain centres have in modulating the incoming sensory activity.

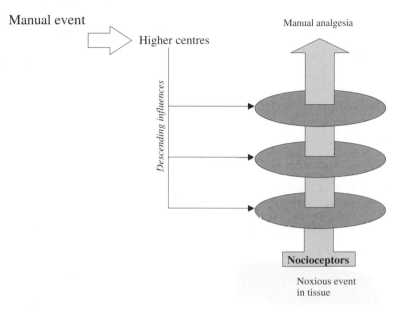

Figure 16.14   Pain relief following manipulation may be related to the potent influences of higher centres in inhibiting noxious afferent signals at different levels within the nervous system.

17

Overview and summary of Section 3

This section has reviewed the response of the whole person to being touched and manipulated. It examined the origins of sensation from the body and its role in the physical and psychological development of the individual. Manipulation has been described as a form of interpersonal communication that can initiate psychological processes. The text on therapeutic manipulation examined the psychodynamic experience of touch and identified two principle forms or aims of manipulation: expressive manipulation, which forms a communication link with the patient and aims to stimulate whole-person well-being and healing, and instrumental manipulation, which aims mechanically to repair the person. Both types of therapeutic intent are important for the treatment of different conditions. In essence, when a condition tends towards the mechanical, instrumental manipulation is appropriate. The use of expressive manipulation is preferred when the patient's condition indicates a psychosomatic causation. However, this does not exclude the concomitant use of both types of manual intent when necessary.

The first chapter of this section was followed by a review of the psychosomatic response and how it is transmitted to the rest of the body. Three pathways were identified: motor, autonomic (parasympathetic and sympathetic) and neuroendocrine. Emotions seem to occur with a patterned response, termed the psychosomatic template, along the three psychosomatic pathways. Manipulation may influence the patterned response by three different thera-peutic modalities: supportive manual therapy, behavioural manual therapy and, as discussed in the previous two Sections, a form of physical therapy.

Overall, this Section encourages the therapist to view the patient as a whole and as an individual of equal standing, which will help the patient during the healing process and elicit a feeling of well-being.

References

1. Muller-Braunschweig H 1986 Psychoanalysis and the body. In: Brahler F (ed) Body experience. Springer-Verlag, London, p 19–34
2. Morris D 1971 Intimate behaviour. Corgi, London
3. Hooker D 1969 The prenatal origin of behavior. Hafner, London
4. Gottlieb G 1971 The oncogenesis of sensory function in birds and mammals. In: Tobach E, Aronson L R, Shaw E (eds) The biopsychology of development. Academic Press, New York
5. Burton A, Heller L G 1964 The touching of the body. Psychoanalytical Review 51: 122–134
6. Bowlby J 1969 Attachment and loss. Hogarth Press, London
7. Parker P 1995 The community children's clinic. Osteopathic Association of Great Britain Newsletter, July, p 7
8. Reite M L 1984 Touch, attachment, and health – is there a relationship? In: Brown C C (ed) The many faces of touch. Johnson & Johnson Baby Products Company Pediatric Round Table Series, 10, p 58–65
9. Schanberg S M, Evoniuk G, Kuhn C M 1984 Tactile and nutritional aspects of maternal care: specific regulators of neuroendocrine function and cellular development. Proceedings of the Society for Experimental Biology and Medicine 175: 135–146
10. Harlow H F 1959 Love in infant monkey. Science. In Physiological Psychology. Thompson R F (ed) W H Freeman, San Francisco, p 78–84
11. Harlow H F 1961 The development of affectional patterns in infant monkeys. In: Foss B M (ed) Determinants of Infant Behaviour. Methuen, London
12. Field et al 1986 Tactile/kinesthetic stimulation effect on preterm neonates. Pediatrics 77(5): 654–658
13. White J L, Labarba R C 1976 The effects of tactile and kinesthetic stimulation on neonatal development in the premature infant. Developmental Psychology 9(6): 569–577
14. Solkoff N, Matuszak D 1975 Tactile stimulation and behavioral development among low-birthweight infants. Child Psychiatry and Human Development 6(1): 33–37
15. Schaeffer J S 1982 The effect of gentle human touch on mechanically ventilated very-short-gestation infants. Maternal Child Nursing Journal, Monograph 12, 11: 4

16. Kattwinkel J, Nearman H S, Fanaroff A A, Katona P G, Klaus M H 1975 Apnea of prematurity: comparative therapeutic effects of cutaneous stimulation and nasal continuous positive airway pressure. Journal of Pediatrics 86: 588–592

17. Wolff G, Money J 1973 Relationship between sleep and growth with reversible somatotropin deficiency (psychological dwarfism). Psychological Medicine 3: 18–27

18. Goodwin D 1978 GCRC research team study link between psycholosocial dwarfism and child abuse. Research Resources Report 2: 1–6

19. Appell G, David M 1961 Case notes on Monique. In: Foss B M (ed). Determinants of infant behaviour. Methuen, London

20. Spitz R 1955 Childhood development phenomena: the influence of the mother–child relationship, and its disturbance. In: Soddy K (ed) Mental health and infant development. Routledge & Kegan Paul, London

21. Spitz R 1955 Childhood development phenomena: the case of Felicia. In: Soddy K (ed) Mental health and infant development. Routledge & Kegan Paul, London

22. Kennell J H 1974 Maternal behavior one year after early and post-partum contact. Developmental Medicine and Child Neurology 16: 172–179

23. Autton N 1989 Touch: an exploration. Darton, Longman & Todd, London

24. Van Wyk J J, Underwood L E 1978 Growth hormone, somatomedins and growth failure. Hospital Care 68: 57–67

25. Lynch J J 1977 The broken heart: the medical consequences of loneliness. Basic Books, New York

26. McAllister F 1995 Marital breakdown and the health of the nation. Copies from 'One plus One', 12 Burlington Street, London W1X 1FF

27. Knapp M L 1977 Nonverbal communication: basic perspectives. In: Stewart J (ed), Bridges not walls: a book about interpersonal communication. Addison-Wesley, London

28. Frank L K 1957 Tactile communication. Genetic Social and General Psychology Monographs 56: 209–255

29. Kulka A, Fry C, Goldstein F J 1960 Kinesthetic needs in infancy. American Journal of Orthopsychiatry 33: 562–571

30. Blauvelt H, McKenna J 1961 Mother–neonate interaction: capacity of the human newborn for orientation. In: Foss B M (ed). Determinants of infant behaviour. Methuen, London

31. Rheingold H L 1961 The effect of environmental stimulation upon social and exploratory behavior in the human infant. In: Foss B M (ed). Determinants of infant behaviour. Methuen, London

32. Stack D M, Muir D W 1992 Adult tactile stimulation during face-to-face interactions modulates five-month-old's affect and attention. Child Development 63(6): 1509–1525

33. Fisher J D, Rytting M, Heslin R 1976 Hands touching hands: affective and evaluative effects of an interpersonal touch. Sociometry 39: 416–421

34. Penny K S 1979 Postpartum perception of touch received during labour. Research in Nursing and Health 2(1): 9–16

35. Farrah S 1971 The nurse the patient and touch. In: Current concepts in clinical nursing. C V Mosby, St Louis

36. Young M 1977 The human touch : who needs it. In: Stewart J (ed) Bridges not walls: a book about interpersonal communication. Addison Wesley, Massachusetts

37. Dominian J 1971 The psychological significance of touch. Nursing Times

38. Pattison J E 1973 Effects of touch on self-exploration and the therapeutic relationship. Journal of Consulting and Clinical Psychology 40(2): 170–175

39. Alagna F J, Whitcher S J, Fisher J D, Wicas E A 1979 Evaluative reaction to interpersonal touch in a counselling interview. Journal of Counselling Psychology 26(6): 465–472

40. McCorkle R 1974 Effects of touch on seriously ill patients. Nursing Research 23(2): 125–132

41. Morales E 1994 Meaning of touch to hospitalized Puerto Ricans with cancer. Cancer Nursing 17(6): 464–469

42. Mercer L S 1966 Touch comfort or threat. Perspectives in Psychiatric Care 4(3): 20–25

43. Fisher J D 1976 Hands touching hands: affective and evaluative effects of an interpersonal touch. Sociometry 39(4): 416–421

44. Patterson M 1976 An arousal model of the inter-personal intimacy. Psychological Review 83: 235–245

45. DeAugustinis J, Isani R A, Ward K F R 1963 Ward study: the meaning of touch in interpersonal communications. In: Burd S, Marshall M (eds) Some clinical approaches to psychiatric nursing. Macmillan, New York

46. Siegal E V 1986 Integrating movement and psychoanalytic technique. In: Robbins A (ed) Expressive therapy. Human Science Press, New York

47. Kepner J I 1993 Body process: working with the body in psychotherapy. Jossey-Bass, San Francisco

48. Clarkson P 1992 Transactional analysis psychotherapy: an integrated approach. Tavistock/Routledge, London

49. Yontef G M 1976 The theory of Gestalt therapy. In: Hatcher C, Himelstein P (eds) The handbook of Gestalt therapy. Jason Aronson, New York

50. Darbonne A 1976 Creative balance: an integration of gestalt, bioenergetics and Rolfing. In: Hatcher C, Himelstein P (eds) The handbook of Gestalt therapy. Jason Aronson, New York

51. Lowen A 1967 The betrayal of the body. Macmillan, London

52. Schilder P 1964 The image and appearance of the human body. John Wiley, Chichester

53. Gorman W 1969 Body image and the image of the brain. Warren H Green, Missouri

54. Rice J B, Hardenbergh M, Hornyak L M 1989 Disturbed body image in anorexia nervosa: dance/movement therapy interventions. In: Hornyak L M, Baker E K (eds) Experiential therapies for eating disorders. Guildford Press, New York

55. Fisher S, Cleveland S E 1968 Body image and personality. Dover Publications, New York

56. Stark A, Aronow S, McGeehan T 1989 Dance/movement therapy with bulimic patients. In: Hornyak L M, Baker E K (eds) Experiential therapies for eating disorders. Guildford Press, New York

57. Nathan B T 1995 Philosophical notes on osteopathy theory. Part II. On persons and bodies, touching and inherent self-healing capacity. British Osteopathic Journal 15: 15–19

58. Weiss SJ 1978 The language of touch: a resource to body image. Issues in Mental Health Nursing 1: 17–29

59. Weiner H 1958 Diagnosis and symptomatology. In: Bellak L (ed) Schizophrenia. Logos Press, New York, p 120, 133–139

60. Kolb L 1959 Disturbances of the body image. In: Arieti S (ed) American handbook of psychiatry. Basic Books, New York, p 749–767

61. Montagu A 1986 Touching: the human significance of the skin. Harper & Row, New York

62. Schopler E 1962 The development of body image and symbol formation through body contact with an autistic child. Journal of Child Psychology 3: 191–202

63. Wilber K 1979 No boundary: eastern and western approaches to personal growth. Shambhala, Boulder, Colorado

64. Cashar L, Dixon B K 1967 The therapeutic use of touch. Journal of Psychiatric Nursing 5: 442–451

65. Roxendal G 1990 Physiotherapy as an approach in psychiatric care with emphasis on body awareness therapy. In: Hegna T, Sveram M (eds) Pychological and psychosomatic problems. Churchill Livingstone, London, p 75–101

66. Sternbach R A 1978 Psychological dimensions and perceptual analysis. In: Carterette E C, Friedman M P (eds) Handbook of perception: feeling and hurting. Academic Press, London, p 231–258

67. Fanslow C A 1984 Touch and the elderly. In: Brown C C (ed) The many faces of touch. Johnson & Johnson Baby Products Company Pediatric Round Table Series, 10, p 183–189

68. Lowen A 1970 Pleasure: a creative approach to life. Penguin Books, New York

69. Lowen A 1975 Bioenergetics. Penguin Books, Harmondsworth

70. In a personal interview with the author to be published at a later date

71. Campbell H J 1973 The pleasure areas. Eyre Methuen, London

72. Hollender M H 1970 The need or wish to be held. Archives of General Psychiatry 22: 445–453

73. Hollender M H, Luborsky L, Scaramella T J 1969 Body contact and sexual enticement. Archives of General Psychiatry 20: 188–191

74. Watson W H 1975 The meaning of touch: geriatric nursing. Journal of Communication 25(3): 104–112

75. Goffman E 1971 Relations in public. Basic Books, New York

76. Weiss S J 1986 Psychophysiological effects of caregiver touch on incidents of cardiac dysrhythmia. Heart and Lung 15(5): 495–505

77. Anderson D 1979 Touching: when is it caring and nurturing or when is it exploitative and damaging? Child Abuse and Neglect 3: 793–794

78. Triplett J L, Arneson S W 1979 The use of verbal and tactile comfort to alleviate distress in young hospitalised children. Research in Nursing and Health 2(1): 17–23

79. Bowlby J 1958 The nature of the child's tie to his mother. International Journal of Psychoanalysis 39: 350–373

80. Nathan B 1995 Philosophical notes on osteopathic theory. Part III. Non-procedural touching and the relationship between touch and emotion. British Osteopathic Journal 17: 31–34

81. Remen N, Blau A A, Hively R 1975 The masculine principle, the feminine principle and humanistic medicine. Institute for the Study of Humanistic Medicine, San Francisco

82. Microsoft encarta 1994

83. Weber R 1984 Philosophers on touch. In: Brown C C (ed) The many faces of touch. Johnson & Johnson Baby Products Company Pediatric Round Table Series, 10, p 3–11

84. Sharaf M 1983 Fury on earth: a biography of Wilhelm Reich. Hutchinson, London

85. Southwell C 1982 Biodynamic massage as a therapeutic tool – with special reference to the biodynamic concept of equilibrium. Journal of Biodynamic Psychology 3: 40–72

86. Bunkan B H, Thornquist E 1990 Psychomotor therapy: an approach to the evaluation and treatment of psychosomatic disorders. In: Hegna T, Sveram M (eds) Pychological and psychosomatic problems. Churchill Livingstone, London, p 45–74

87. MacLean P D 1970 The triune brain, emotion and scientific bias. In: Schmitt F O (ed) Neuroscience: second study program. Rockefeller University Press, New York

88. Guyton A G 1991 Textbook of physiology. W B Saunders, Philadelphia

89. Kelly D H W 1980 Anxiety and emotions: physiological basis and treatment. Charles C Thomas, Springfield, IL

90. Abrahams V C, Hilton S M, Zbrozyna A 1960 Active muscle vasodilatation produced by stimulation of the brain stem: its significance in the defense reaction. Journal of Physiology 154: 491

91. Balshan I D 1962 Muscle tension and personality in women. Archives of General Psychiatry 7: 436–448

92. Schwartz G E, Fair P L, Mandel M R, Salt P S, Mieske M, Klerman G L 1978 Facial electromyography in the assessment of improvement in depression. Psychosomatic Medicine 40: 4

93. Gellhorn E 1964 Motion and emotion: the role of proprioception in the physiology and pathophysiology of the emotions. Psychological Review 71(6): 457–472

94. von Euler C, Sonderberg U 1958 Co-ordinated changes in temperature thresholds for thermoregulatory reflexes. Acta Physiologica Scandinavica 42: 112–129

95. Ban T, Masai H, Sakai A, Kurotsu T 1951 Experimental studies on sleep by the electrical stimulation of the hypothalamus. Medical Journal, Osaka University 2: 145–161

96. French J D 1972 The reticular formation. In: Physiological psychology, W H Freeman, San Francisco

97. Blair D A, Glover W E, Greenfield A D M, Roddie I C 1959 Excitation of cholinergic vasodilator nerves to human skeletal muscles during emotional stress. Journal of Physiology 148: 633–647

98. Lynch J J et al 1974 The effects of human contact on cardiac arrhythmia in coronary care patients. Journal of Nervous and Mental Disease 158: 2

99. Gantt W H, Newton J E O, Royer F L, Stephens J H 1966 Effects of person. Conditional Reflexes 1: 18–35

100. Lynch J J, Flaherty L, Emrich C, Mills M E, Katcher A 1974 Effects of human contact on heart activity of curarized patients. American Heart Journal 88(2): 160–169

101. Geis F, Viksne V 1972 Touching: physical contact and level of arousal. Proceedings of the 80th Annual Convention of the American Psychological Association 7: 179–180

102. Willoughby J O, Martin J B 1978 The role of the limbic system in neuroendocrine regulation. In: Livingston K E, Hornykiewicz O (eds) Limbic mechanisms. Plenum Press, London

103. Mason J W 1968 A review of psychoendocrine research on the pituitary–adrenal cortical system. Psychosomatic Medicine 30: 576

104. Mason J W 1968 A review of psychoendocrine research on the sympathetic-adrenal medullary system. Psychosomatic Medicine 30: 631

105. Levine S 1972 Stress and behavior. In: Physiological psychology. W H Freeman, San Francisco

106. Levi L 1965 The urinary output of adrenaline and noradrenaline during different experimentally induced pleasant and unpleasant emotional states. Psychosomatic Medicine 27: 80

107. Curruthers M, Taggart P 1973 Vagotonicity of violence: biochemical and cardiac responses to violent films and television programmes. British Medical Journal 3: 384

108. Levi L 1969 Sympathoadrenomedullary activity, diuresis, and emotional reactions during visual sexual stimulation in human females and males. Psychosomatic Medicine 31: 251

109. Handelson J H et al 1962 Psychological factors lowering plasma 17-hydroxycorticosteroids concentration. Psychosomatic Medicine 24: 535

110. Raab W 1971 Cardiotoxic biochemical effects of emotional-environmental stressors – fundamentals of psychocardiology. In: Levi L (ed) Society stress and disease. Oxford University Press, London

111. Sachar E J, Baron M 1979 The biology of affective disorders. Annual Review of Neuroscience 2: 505–518

112. Barker J C 1968 Scared to death. An examination of fear, its causes and effects. Frederick Muller, London

113. Kelly D H W 1966 Measurements of anxiety by forearm blood flow. British Journal of Psychiatry 112: 789

114. Sachar E J, Fishman J R, Mason J W 1965 Influence of hypnotic trance on plasma 17-hydroxycorticosteroids concentration. Psychosomatic Medicine 27: 330

115. Barr J S, Taslitz N 1970 The influence of back massage on autonomic function. Physical Therapy 60: 1679–1691

116. Schmidt R F, Schonfuss K 1970 An analysis of the reflex activity in the cervical sympathetic trunk induced by myelinated somatic afferents. Pflugers Archives 314: 175–198

117. McDougall J 1989 Theatres of the body: a psychoanalytical approach to psychosomatic illness. Free Association Books, London

118. Kuntz A 1945 Anatomic and physiologic properties of cutaneo-visceral vasomotor reflex arcs. Journal of Neurophysiology 8: 421–430

119. Sato A, Kaufman A, Koizumi K, Brooks C 1969 Afferent nerve groups and sympathetic reflex pathways. Brain Research 14: 575–587

120. Sato A, Schmidt R F 1973 Somatosympathetic reflexes. Afferent fibres, central pathways and discharge characteristics. Physiological Reviews 53: 916–947

121. Denny-Brown D 1968 Motor mechanisms – introduction: the general principle of motor integration. In: Field J, Magoun H W, Hall V E (eds) Handbook of physiology, Section 1, Volume 2. Williams & Wilkins, Baltimore, p 781–796

122. Ganong W F 1981 Review of medical physiology, 10th edn. Lange, California

123. Cannon W B, Rosenblueth A 1949 The supersensitivity of denervated structures. Macmillan, New York

124. Rushmer R F, Smith O A, Lasher E P 1960 Neural mechanisms of cardiac control during exertion. Physiological Reviews 40(4): 27

125. Sherrington C S 1906 The integrative action of the nervous system. Yale University Press, New Haven, CT

126. Heymans C, Neil E 1958 Reflexogenic areas of the cardiovascular system. J & A Churchill, London

127. Folkow B 1956 Nervous control of the blood vessels. In: McDowell R J S (ed) The control of the circulation of the blood. W M Dawson, London

128. Darwin C 1872, 1934 The expression of the emotions in man and animal. Watts, London

129. Cohen M J, Rickles W H, McArthur D L 1978 Evidence for physiological response stereotype in migraine headache. Psychosomatic Medicine 40(4): 344–354

130. Munro A 1972 Psychosomatic medicine. I. The psychosomatic approach. Practitioner 208: 162–168

131. Sartory G, Lader M 1981 Psychophysiology and drugs in anxiety and phobias. In: Christie M J, Mellett P G (eds) Foundations of psychosomatics. John Wiley, New York, ch 8, p 169–221

132. Steptoe A 1986 Psychophysiological contributions to the understanding and management of essential hypertension. In: Christie M J, Mellett P G (eds) The psychosomatic approach: contemporary practice of whole-person care. John Wiley, New York, p 171–189

133. Reiser M F, Bakst H 1959 Psychology of cardiovascular disorders. In: Arieti S (ed) American handbook of psychiatry. Basic Books, New York, p 659–677

134. Lidz T 1959 General concepts of psychosomatic medicine. In: Arieti S (ed) American handbook of psychiatry. Basic Books, New York, p 647–658

135. Plotnik R, Mollenauer S 1978 Brain and behavior. Canefield Press, London

136. DeLongis A, Coyne J C, Dakof G, Folkman S, Lazarus R S 1982 Relationship of daily hassles, uplifts, and major life events to health status. Health Psychology 1(2): 119–136

137. Dixon N F 1981 Psychosomatic disorder: a special case of subliminal perception. In: Christie M J, Mellett P G (eds) Foundations of psychosomatics. John Wiley, New York

138. Cook E, Christie M J, Gartshore S, Stern R M, Venables P H 1981 After the executive monkey. In: Christie M J, Mellett P G (eds) Foundations of psychosomatics. John Wiley, New York, ch 11, p 245–258

139. Reich W 1933, 1991 Character analysis. Noonday Press, New York

140. Stewart I, Joines V. Today: a new introduction to T.A. Lifespace Publishing

141. Keleman S 1981 Your body speaks its mind. Centre Press, Berkeley, CA

142. Levey A B, Martin I 1981The relevance of classical conditioning to psychosomatic disorders. In: Christie M J, Mellett P G (eds) Foundations of psychosomatics. John Wiley, New York, ch 12, p 259–282

143. Freeman G L 1948 The energetics of human behavior. Cornell University Press, Ithaca, New York

144. Adamec R E 1978 Normal and abnormal limbic system mechanisms of emotive biasing. In: Livingston K E, Hornykiewicz O (eds) Limbic mechanisms. Plenum Press, New York, pp 405–455

145. Schawarz S P, Blanchard E B 1986 Behavioral treatment of irritable bowel syndrome: a 1-year follow-up study. Biofeedback and Self-Regulation 11(3): 189–198

146. Radnitz C L, Blanchard E B 1989 A 1- and 2-year follow-up study of bowel sound biofeedback as a treatment for irritable bowel syndrome. Biofeedback and Self-regulation 14(4): 333–338

147. McCroskery J H, Engel B T 1981 Biofeedback and emotional behaviour. In: Christie M J, Mellett P G (eds) Foundations of psychosomatics. John Wiley, New York, p 193–221

148. Lederman E 1997 Harmonic technique. Churchill Livinstone, Edinburgh (in press)

149. Gordon T , Foss B M 1966 The role of stimulation in the delay of onset of crying in the newborn infant. Quarterly Journal of Experimental Psychology 18: 79–81

150. Korner A F, Thoman E B 1972 The relative efficacy of contact and vestibular-proprioceptive stimulation in soothing neonates. Child Development 43: 443–453

151. Ayers A J 1979 Sensory integration and learning disorders. Weston Psychological Services, Los Angeles

152. Casler L 1965 The effect of extra tactile stimulation on a group of institutionalized infants. Genetic Social and General Psychological Monographs 71: 137–175

153. Korner A F, Guilleminault C, Van den Hoed J, Baldwin R B 1978 Reduction of sleep apnea and bradycardia in preterm infants on oscillating water beds: a controlled polygraphic study. Pediatrics 61(4): 528–533

154. Rausch P B 1984 A tactile and kinesthetic stimulation program for premature infants. In: Brown C C (ed) The many faces of touch. Johnson & Johnson Baby Products Company Pediatric Round Table Series, 10, p 101–106

155. Korner A F 1984 The many faces of touch. In: Brown C C (ed) The many faces of touch. Johnson & Johnson Baby Products Company Pediatric Round Table Series, 10, p 107–113

156. Korner A F, Schneider P 1983 Effects of vestibular-proprioceptive stimulation on the neurobehavioral development of preterm infants: a pilot study. Neuropediatrics 14: 170–175

157. Elton D 1987 Emotion variables and chronic pain management. Elsevier, Amsterdam

158. Korr I M 1947 Neuronal basis of the osteopathic lesion. Journal of the American Osteopathic Association 47: 191–198

159. Wright A 1995 Hypoalgesia post-manipulative therapy: a review of a potential neurophysiological mechanism. Manual Therapy 1: 11–16

160. Casey K L 1978 Neural mechanisms of pain. In: Carterette E C, Friedman M P (eds) Handbook of perception: feeling and hurting. Academic Press, London, p 183–219

161. Fetz E E 1968 Pyramidal tract effects on interneurones in the cat lumbar dorsal horn. Journal of Neurophysiology 31: 69–80

162. Andersen P, Eccles J C, Sears T A 1964 Cortically evoked depolarization of primary afferent fibres in the spinal cord. Journal of Neurophysiology 27: 63–77

163. Reynolds D G 1969 Surgery in the rat during electrical analgesia induced by focal brain stimulation. Science 164: 444–445

164. Richardson D E 1976 Brain stimulation for pain control. IEEE Transactions on Biomedical Engineering 23: 304–306

Overview and clinical application

18

Overview and clinical application

This book is a study and search for the physiological, neurological and psychophysiological basis of manual therapy. To understand the effect that manipulation has on the patient, a physiological model of manipulation has been proposed. In this model, the responses of the individual to manipulation are seen to occur at three levels of organization: local tissue, neurological and psychophysiological. Each of these is a source of unique physiological responses. Many treatment outcomes can be attributed to the stimulation of one or more of these organizations by manipulation.

Local tissue organization

At this level, the effect of manipulation is on:

- tissue repair processes
- the structural and biomechanical behaviour of the tissue
- tissue fluid dynamics.

Techniques affecting the different processes have been identified and correlated with common clinical conditions. Those conditions related to the local tissue organization have been classified as being 'solid' or 'soft'. Solid conditions are those in which tissue morphology and structure have altered, for example in contractures, adhesions, lack of extendibility and loss of range of movement. These are mostly affected by tensile techniques such as stretching and deep massage. The aim of these techniques is to promote a change in the structure and mechanical behaviour of the tissue. Soft conditions are those in which the local extracellular environment has changed as a result of injury or pathological processes, leading, for example, to oedema, inflammation or joint effusion. These conditions are more effectively treated by rhythmic, intermittent compression, pump-like techniques and movement, the aim of which is to encourage fluid flow between the interstitial, lymph and blood plasma fluid compartments. This movement of fluid will ultimately influence the cellular environment, resulting in changes in the internal cellular compartment and affecting cellular processes. Manipulation may influence cellular metabolic activity, health and viability.

Neurological organization

The section examining the neurological organization of the motor system put forward the argument that functional organization is more important than structural organization in rehabilitating the motor system. Manual techniques which may influence the motor system have been identified and their effect on proprioception discussed. Proprioceptors only provide feedback and cannot control the motor system. Motor outcome is brought about by centrifugal, central processes. It means that manipulation cannot be used to control the motor system, and that the use of manipulation in rehabilitation should be in a form of guidance. It was established that active techniques in which there is cognition and volition on the side of the patient are the most effective in producing long-term adaptation. Reflexive or passive types of treatment have little or no effect on motor processes. The use of active techniques in relation to various motor system and musculoskeletal conditions has been discussed. Areas in which manual guidance can be used for the neurological organization are:

- postural and movement guidance
- neuromuscular rehabilitation following musculoskeletal injuries
- rehabilitation of the motor system following central nervous damage.

Since rehabilitation of these different conditions involves motor learning and adaptation processes, the principles of guidance are fairly comparable in the treatment of different musculoskeletal and motor conditions.

Psychophysiological organization

At the level of psychophysiological organization, it was demonstrated how touch 'moves the mind' – the psychodynamics of manipulation. This section began by looking at manipulation as a sensory experience and how it initiates different psychological processes. It showed manipulation to be a form of interpersonal communication, and discussed its effects on the body-self (or body-mind), and manipulation as a therapeutic process. This was followed by examining how psychological processes are transmitted and expressed in the body via three physiological pathways: the motor system, the autonomic system and the neuroendocrine system. Because these pathways control every biological process in the body, the physiological response is a total body response, not restricted to one organ, tissue or system. This physiological outcome is unpredictable as far as which systems will benefit from the effects of manipulation. Therefore, treatment cannot be directed towards single organs or tissues, for example the heart or the gut. Physiological changes in these organs and systems come about by the total reduction in arousal that may follow manual treatment. General physiological changes that may occur at this level are:

- general muscle relaxation
- generalized altered visceral activity
- altered pain perception.

It must be noted that these physiological changes are only possibilities, potentials which may or may not be fulfilled in response to treatment. The three pathways to the soma are the origins of the concept of psychosomatic templates, in which emotion is supported by stereotypic somatic patterns. Three roles for manipulation have been identified in influencing the psychosomatic response: manual therapy as supportive, behavioural and physical therapy. In its supportive role, manual therapy may help to reduce anxiety and stress, which may be the aetiology of the presenting somatic condition. In its behavioural role, manual therapy can be used to guide the patient to postural and movement patterns that reduce mechanical stress on the musculoskeletal system. Where specific areas of the musculoskeletal system are held in tension, the patient can be guided in how to relax these areas. At the end of the psychosomatic sequence, at the tissue organization, manual therapy can help to improve health status and functional ability, and initiate a structural change. This may help tissue to cope better under conditions of stress and increased demand.

At the psychosomatic organization, manipulation provides unique physical contact, an environment in which whole-person healing/reparative processes and well-being are supported. The potency of such interaction is derived from the instinctive needs and regressive processes of the individual.

IMITATING NATURE'S WAY

Much of the content of this book considers the search for the body's reparative and healing mechanisms, understanding how the body 'does it naturally' and offering a manual support for these physiological mechanisms. Indeed, many of the manual techniques described imitate and amplify healing processes. For example, on a local tissue level, manual techniques can imitate the natural mechanical stresses that direct fibroblasts and collagen alignment in the connective tissue matrix and muscle, including the orientation of the muscle cells. At the neurological organization, manipulation imitates natural motor learning sequences, facilitating neuromuscular adaptation.

MANUAL THERAPY AS A STIMULUS FOR ADAPTATION

Manual therapy can be seen as a stimulus for adaptation in the body. The physical interaction between the therapist and the patient provides a new situation to which the patient's body has to adapt. For example, a muscle that is shortened from postural or traumatic causes comprises a form of adaptation but may fail to meet the challenges of daily demands. A treatment that uses stretching to elongate the muscle is forcing the muscle to re-adapt to a new experience (Fig. 18.1). A successful treatment is one in which the adaptation to treatment has been transferred to daily or leisure activities. In the example of the shortened muscle, its lengthening adaptation to treatment allows the individual to walk or sit with reduced mechanical stress and discomfort.

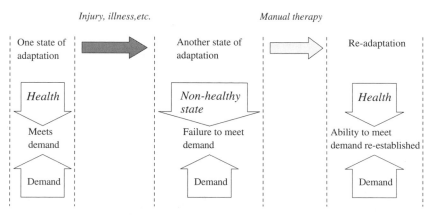

Figure 18.1   Manual therapy as facilitating an adaptive process.

Another important treatment principle identified is that adaptation is a highly specific process, i.e. the body learns and performs best the activity that has been practised. For example, if the reparative process is allowed to progress with a background of immobility, the healed tissue will not perform well under conditions of movement or mechanical stress. Tissues that heal under conditions of movement are well adapted to movement when the individual returns to daily activity. Adaptation goes beyond local tissue events, similar processes also being present in the neuromuscular connections. Here, too, the adaptation process is highly specific, and the system will adapt and perform effectively the guided activity provided during rehabilitation. Treatment that encourages an adaptation process similar to normal functional activity will transfer well to the individual's life.

Overall, manual therapy can be seen as directing and facilitating the body's own repair and adaptive processes.

MANUAL TOOLS

Manual techniques are the professional tools of the manual therapist. To some extent, manual tools have a definite physical shape in the form of the changing shape of the therapist's hand: changes in mechanical leverage, contact area, amplitude of force, etc. Their influence is not limited to their physical shape, but also involves their pattern of application and the therapist's intention.

One can visualize an imaginary cabinet in which different manual techniques are stored, to be picked and chosen according to the patient's condition or needs (Fig. 18.2). Each technique group has a characteristic physiological affect, each with its strength and weakness at the different organizational levels. Some techniques are potent at stimulating fluid flow, others are potent at stretching muscle and others, with the right intent, may have a potent influence on the patient's mind. A large cabinet with a wealth of techniques will help to increase the spectrum of conditions the therapist is able to treat.

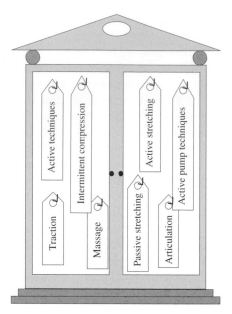

Figure 18.2   The manual tools cabinet.

CRITERIA OF TECHNIQUES NEEDED TO INFLUENCE THE THREE ORGANIZATIONS

Different groups of technique have strengths and weaknesses for the different organizations. Some will be more effective for one organization, but this potency may be severely reduced at other levels. This would imply the use of alternative rather than ineffective techniques. There are certain 'physiological rules' or criteria that the manual technique must obey in order to influence each of the three organizations (Fig 18.3).

Criteria for local tissue organization

The hallmark of techniques at this level is that they must be able mechanically to load the tissue and deform it. They must either produce joint movement (e.g. articulation or joint oscillation), rhythmically deform the tissue to promote fluid flow changes (e.g. massage, effleurage or intermittent compression) or have the correct amplitude and force to be able to cause permanent elongation of shortened tissue (e.g. passive and active stretches).

Nature of manipulation

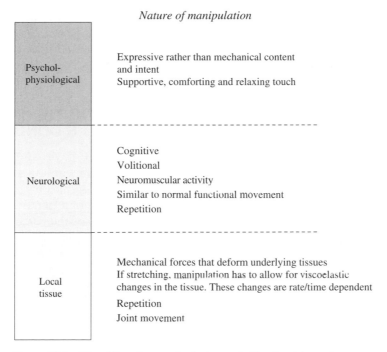

Psychol-physiological	Expressive rather than mechanical content and intent Supportive, comforting and relaxing touch
Neurological	Cognitive Volitional Neuromuscular activity Similar to normal functional movement Repetition
Local tissue	Mechanical forces that deform underlying tissues If stretching, manipulation has to allow for viscoelastic changes in the tissue. These changes are rate/time dependent Repetition Joint movement

Figure 18.3 The different manual criteria needed to stimulate each organization effectively.

Repetition is another important character that techniques for this level must have. Tissue repair processes depend on repetitive mechanical activity for normal tissue architecture and mechanical behaviour, for example cycles of passive and active technique. Similarly, fluid dynamics are largely affected by rhythmic activity that occurs over many cycles. Stretching shortened tissue is also dependent not only on repetition, but also on the length of time the tissue is stretched. The longer that time, the greater and more permanent the changes will be. Transient and singular manual events will be ineffective at influencing processes on the local tissue level.

Criteria for neurological organization

To be able to influence this organization, manipulation must have several characteristics. Foremost, it must be cognitive and volitional. The patient must be actively involved in the manipulation. There must be muscle activity that is initiated centrally: the motor system is very 'resilient' to passive techniques or reflexive treatment initiated from the periphery.

Repetition is also important at the level of the neurological organization. Movement patterns have to be repeated many times for long-term adaptation to take place. Short, transient and singular events are unlikely to initiate an adaptive response in the nervous system. Furthermore, the manual event must be similar to normal functional movement: the closer the manual pattern is to daily patterns, the greater the potential that this movement will transfer to daily activities. Movement that is non-physiological or non-functional will fail to transfer to normal daily use.

Techniques that meet these criteria are the different active techniques such as movement and postural guidance and neuromuscular rehabilitation.

Criteria for psychophysiological organization

This organization holds a paradox. Since touch is a psychodynamic event, manipulation will, regardless of its mechanical content, affect this level. However, the potency of this effect lies in the expressive nature of the physical interaction between therapist and patient, rather than in the mechanical content or form of the technique. It implies that treatment that is highly mechanistic and detached may fail to meet the patient psychologically.

Efficacy of treatment is related to the ability of the therapist to communicate through touch, messages of support, comfort and compassion, and to the ability of the patient to comprehend these messages. Techniques at this level have no true form but, like other forms of interpersonal communication, reflect interactions between two individuals, the effects of manipulation being related to the whole treatment event rather than a specific technique. At this level, one can only speak of 'manual events' rather than specific manual techniques.

CORRELATING TECHNIQUE WITH THE PATIENT'S CONDITION

In Table 18.1, I have attempted to correlate different manual techniques with some common musculoskeletal conditions often seen in my own practice. This is not a treatment recipe but rather a demonstration of the correlation process I use; it is only a limited example of a full treatment. A full treatment usually has non-manual elements such as exercise instruction and ergonomic advice. Elements of treatment that are outside the scope of this book are not included in Table 18.1.

Table 18.1   Correlating common clinical conditions with manual techniques. This is not a treatment recipe but an example of a possible correlation process. Each patient and his or her condition is unique, and treatment must be designed to suit each patient's needs. This table does not represent a full treatment, but only the manual portion of the whole therapeutic event. Text in bold denotes the organizational level where the main treatment drive may be everted.

Condition	Local tissue (Section 1)	Neurological (Section 2)	Psychophysiological (Section 3)
Muscle strain and inflammation (e.g. spinal muscle injury after lifting)	*Aim*: **Initially, support repair process and improve flow. Later, improve tissue extendibility by stretching** *Possible techniques*: **Initially, intermittent compression and massage techniques. Later, with improvement in tensile strength, add gentle, cyclical stretching**	If muscle wasting is present, improve neuromuscular activity using different motor abilities Use active techniques to rehabilitate the neuromuscular link	
Muscle ischaemia (e.g. due to compartment syndrome)	*Aim*: **Improve flow within muscle. Reduce any impediment to flow** *Possible techniques*: **To improve flow, use both passive and active muscle pump techniques. To reduce impediment to flow, use stretching techniques (e.g. longitudinal, cross-fibre and active stretching techniques)**	As above, but may also need to work on movement and postural pattern that may underlie compartment syndrome	
Soft-tissue shortening	*Aim*: **Improve extendibility of soft tissue** *Possible techniques*: **Active and passive stretch techniques**	If due to central nervous damage, will need to stimulate neuromuscular connection (see below) If postural aetiology, work with postural guidance	

Table 18.1 (*contd*)

Condition	Local tissue (Section 1)	Neurological (Section 2)	Psychophysiological (Section 3)
Joint inflammation and effusion (e.g. facet, ankle or knee joint strain)	*Aim*: **Initially, support repair process and improve fluid flow in and out of joint cavity. Later, increase joint range of movement** *Possible techniques*: **Initially, joint articulation, oscillation and movement, all within pain-free range. Later, increase range by passive stretching techniques**	If muscle wasting is present, stimulate neuromuscular connection, working with active–dynamic techniques and abilities Immediately after injury, active techniques may cause further irritation. Need to wait until inflammation and pain are reduced before working at this level	
Articular damage (e.g. post-fracture, arthritis, etc.)	**As above**	As above	
Adhesive capsulitis (e.g. frozen shoulder)	**As above**	As above	
Disc damage	**As above, but strong stretching may be left out**	As above	
Nerve root irritation	*Aim*: **Initially, support repair process at site of irritation, improve fluid flow and reduce swelling** *Possible techniques*: **Rhythmic, cyclical spinal articulation. Use cycles of flexion/extension, side-bending or rotation within the pain-free range, work only with articulation patterns that reduce the symptoms**	As above	
Abnormal motor tone due to central motor damage (e.g. stroke, palsies, etc.)	**If, due to inflammation or ischaemia, musculoskeletal pain is present, use techniques described above to improve flow** **If contractures are present, use techniques described for 'soft-tissue shortening'**	*Aim*: **Re-establish communication within motor system. Support repair and adaptation** *Possible techniques*: **If spasticity is present, reduce by inhibitory techniques or use motor relaxation techniques** **Re-establish lost motor abilities by guiding patient using cognitive and volitional movement** **If patient is unable to initiate movement, use passive guidance initially. Once patient is capable of moving voluntarily, use active techniques**	Patient likely to be emotionally distressed. Use comforting and supportive touch Re-establish body image by working on the skin with massage and stroking-type techniques To stimulate deep proprioception, use passive movements and active techniques (if possible) Can use passive movement to increase awareness and connection with dysfunctional part of the body
Muscle wasting due to joint injury		*Aim*: **Re-establish normal neuromuscular activity and reduce arthrogenic inhibition.** *Possible techniques*: **Active–dynamic techniques within motor abilities spectrum**	
Post-injury functional instability in joints (e.g. following ankle sprains)		As above	

Table 18.1 (*contd*)

Condition	Local tissue (Section 1)	Neurological (Section 2)	Psychophysiological (Section 3)
Abnormal posture and movement	**If full potential of posture is limited by tissue shortening, use active and passive stretching to improve range and ease of movement**	*Aim:* **Motor learning of more 'correct' postural and movement patterns** *Possible techniques:* **Postural guidance which is similar to normal movement**	**Increase awareness of posture by working on superficial proprioception using broad massage and stroking Work on deep proprioception using articulation techniques and active techniques Work with patient on psychopostural part of body image**
General increase in muscle tone (from anxiety and stress)	If arousal state is chronic, there may be structural changes in muscles. May need to elongate shortened muscles by active and passive stretching, or reduce ischaemic pain by use of passive and active pump techniques	**Use motor relaxation techniques**	*Aim:* **Reduce arousal** *Possible techniques:* **Supportive and comforting manipulation. Use of expressive touch rather than mechanical approach**
Local increase in muscle tone due to patterns of holding and expression	If long term, local changes may be present in muscle. May need to elongate shortened muscles by active and passive stretching, or reduce ischaemic pain by use of passive and active pump techniques	**Use motor relaxation techniques**	*Aim:* **Guide a change in psychosomatic behaviour that will reduce overactivity in designated muscle group**

PAIN RELIEF BY MANIPULATION

Pain commonly determines the beginning and the termination of treatment. It is usually pain that motivates the patient to seek help, and the alleviation of pain that will mark the end of most treatments. Although in manual therapy the stated aim is to remove the causes of the patient's condition, reducing pain often takes precedence. Unless pain symptoms are immediately addressed, it is very likely that patients will seek pain relief elsewhere. It is often difficult to motivate patients who are pain-free to return to treatments that may help them in the long term.

There may be several mechanisms underlying pain relief during manipulation (Fig. 18.4), local mechanisms of which were reviewed in Section 1. It is proposed that some pain relief following treatment is related to the effects of manipulation on fluid dynamics at the site of damage. Increasing the flow and reducing swelling may lead to a decrease in chemical and mechanical irritation at the site of inflammation. Section 2 reviewed possible neurological mechanisms for manually induced pain relief (manual analgesia). Pain relief may be due to sensory gating of noxious sensation by activation of proprioceptors. Section 3 reviewed the psychological mechanism of manually induced analgesia. It highlighted the importance of higher centres in influencing the perception of pain. Psychologically, pain may initiate a process of fragmentation of the body image. Reducing pain is therefore important for body image reintegration. Evoking a sense of pleasure in the painful area may also help to facilitate the integration processes.

The model proposed here for pain relief by manipulation does not comprise a total treatment. Full pain management needs to take into consideration non-manual elements such as posture, psychosocial elements, emotion and the physical environment of the patient.

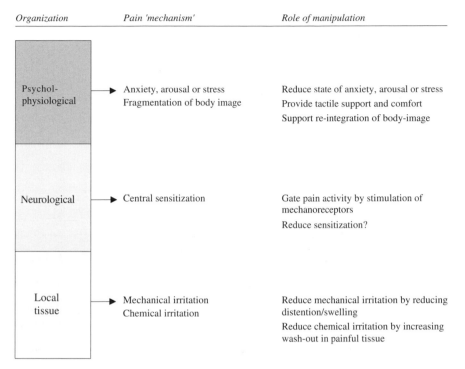

Figure 18.4   The possible role of manipulation in providing pain relief.

Index